Coaching the Rider
Theory and Practice

Jane Houghton Brown
FBHS

b

**Blackwell
Science**

© Jane Houghton Brown and
Sarah Pilliner 1995
Blackwell Science Ltd
Editorial Offices:
Osney Mead, Oxford OX2 0EL
25 John Street, London WC1N 2BL
23 Ainslie Place, Edinburgh EH3 6AJ
238 Main Street, Cambridge
  Massachusetts 02142, USA
54 University Street, Carlton
  Victoria 3053, Australia

Other Editorial Offices:
Arnette Blackwell SA
  1, rue de Lille, 75007 Paris
France

Blackwell Wissenschafts-Verlag GmbH
  Kurfürstendamm 57
  10707 Berlin, Germany

  Feldgasse 13, A-1238 Wien
  Austria

First published 1995

Set in 11pt Times
by DP Photosetting, Aylesbury, Bucks
Printed and bound in Great Britain
at the Alden Press Limited,
Oxford and Northampton

DISTRIBUTORS

Marston Book Services Ltd
PO Box 87
Oxford OX2 0DT
(*Orders:* Tel: 01865 791155
        Fax: 01865 791927
        Telex: 837515)

USA
  Blackwell Science Inc.
  238 Main Street
  Cambridge, MA 02142
  (*Orders:* Tel: 800 215-1000
          617 876 7000
        Fax: 617 492-5263)

Canada
  Oxford University Press
  70 Wynford Drive
  Don Mills
  Ontario M3C 1J9
  (*Orders:* Tel: 416 441 2941)

Australia
  Blackwell Science Pty Ltd
  54 University Street
  Carlton, Victoria 3053
  (*Orders:* Tel: 03 347-0300
        Fax: 03 349-3016)

A catalogue record for this title
is available from the British Library

ISBN 0–632–03931–0

Library of Congress
Cataloging-in-Publication Data

Brown, Jane Houghton.
    Coaching the rider : theory and practice/
Jane Houghton Brown.
        p.   cm.
    Includes index.
        ISBN 0–632–03931–0 (pbk. : alk. paper)
        1. Horsemanship—Study and teaching.
I. Title.
SF310.5.B76   1995
798.2′3′071—dc20   95-662
                                    CIP

Contents

Preface

This book clearly explains how to teach riding and how to coach competitors. Modern techniques of teaching riders have their roots in the tried and tested methods of the old cavalry schools, which have been refined for use in civilian life in riding schools and the Pony Club. This century there has been great growth in competitive riding at all levels and with this has arrived the new techniques of competitive coaching.

Also there has suddenly blossomed a great openness of teaching and coaching from one country to another; this book is the first to include this breadth of understanding which has brought a new freedom from some of the set ways and dogma while encouraging high standards in achievement and understanding.

For all who seek to instruct, teach better or to coach, be it at novice or primary standard or right across the spectrum to international level, this book provides essential knowledge. Those who wish to become riding instructors, and possibly take ascending examinations to prove their skills, need to be familiar with the techniques and understanding which are clearly shown in this book. Those who seek to help competitors owe it to those competitors and their horses to ensure that their coaching is soundly based, not only in what they teach but how they teach it.

My inspiration to write this book has come from my close involvement with young instructors who have often bemoaned the lack of written guidance on this fascinating subject. The experiences of a decade of competing at high levels in a range of disciplines, together with 25 years of teaching, have been stored in my mind and I feel a real desire to share these experiences with others. This book examines the hitherto neglected area of teaching theory, backed up by extensive practical examples, many of which stem from personal experience.

I have been fortunate enough to have been taught by leading trainers, including Colonel Jo Hume Dudgeon and Franz Rochawanski, and I would like to pay tribute to them all. I am sure that my own teaching reflects my interpretation of their philosophies and it is a privilege to be able to share these philosophies.

My motivation when teaching is to try to ensure that everybody involved benefits: the horses by enhancing their performance through physical well-being and mental stability; the riders by stretching their minds and bodies whilst developing their technical skills; and the coaches by keeping an open, enquiring mind whilst giving themselves entirely to each pupil they teach. My philosophy is summed up by Charles Dickens, who wrote:

'Whatever I have tried to do in my life;
I have tried with all my heart to do it well.
Whatever I have devoted myself to, I have devoted
myself completely; in aims great and small, I have
always been thoroughly in earnest'

Having read this book, no doubt there will be many areas where you could say 'I do all this already', but what I hope you will also say is that 'this book has provoked a great deal of thought, it has helped me to refresh my teaching and above all to "accentuate the positive and eliminate the negative"'.

Acknowledgements

The author would like to thank Sarah Pilliner for all her hard work and effort putting the words into readable order and putting the whole thing on disk. Thanks also to Clive Milkins for his help on teaching riders with disabilities. Finally, thanks to her husband Jeremy for his patience and understanding.

Part I
Effective Teaching

1 Training and Coaching

Who is a trainer? Well, really anyone who trains anybody to do anything and, in theory, the principles of training remain the same whatever the technicalities involved.

We in the equine industry undoubtedly have a weakness in this particular sphere. We have traditionally taught people to conduct a lesson by:

- having control of the situation, in other words the horse and rider plus associated safety aspects;
- making observations about the horse's way of going and the rider's influence on him, including the aids and rider position;
- correcting the faults as they arise;
- summing up and giving some homework.

Well, what is wrong with that, you might ask. Nothing, as far as it goes *but* it could go a good deal further, encompassing and enhancing the methods outlined above.

Qualities of a good trainer

Motivation
Trainers must be motivated – they must want to train. They must ask themselves 'Why do I want to train?'. Perhaps they find the possibility that they can improve another person's performance by sharing their knowledge and experience quite fascinating.

A key factor for many is concern for the horse. The acquisition of any knowledge or skill that enables the horse to perform with minimum mental and physical stress is of vital importance.

It is also vital for the future to train the trainer so that the overall standard of teaching and coaching in the horse industry is comparable with other sports.

Training people to win has not been mentioned and some of you may feel this to be your main aim or ambition. Certainly it is satisfying to train winners but it should not be top of the list. In just the same way it is questionable whether people should be trained specifically for examination; it is more beneficial in the long run to train people to perform with skill and understanding so that they are useful to the industry and by coincidence will probably pass exams.

Knowledge
Trainers must be knowledgeable. They have a responsibility to study and keep up-to-date with the specific requirements of the equine discipline that their pupils are involved in.

Credibility
Trainers must either be skilled enough to demonstrate effectively or have a proven track record in order for them to be able to command the respect of pupils.

Honesty
Trainers must be honest with both themselves and their pupils. This may well mean having to tackle parents, owners and sponsors when evaluating the likelihood of a goal not being achievable. There are so many players in our particular field and getting them all to work together as a team is one of our hardest tasks. We have a tendency to be parochial and, even worse, to run each other down. It is rarely beneficial, but if we are honest with ourselves, we are probably all guilty from time to time. We may see it as evaluating the situation but the trainer must take care to remain objective.

Communication
The trainer must be a good communicator (Fig. 1.1). Communication is the vital link that enables all the principles of good training to be used to best advantage. We often say that the trainer/teacher/ instructor must have a well modulated clear voice; this is very true, and especially so when teaching in a one-to-one situation. In small groups where sound carries well, encourage the pupils to listen by speaking in as normal a way as possible. More important than the voice is empathy – the ability to relate to your pupils. Try to get inside them and feel for them; are they nervous, happy, confident or confused? If a natural feeling does not flow across, then talk to your

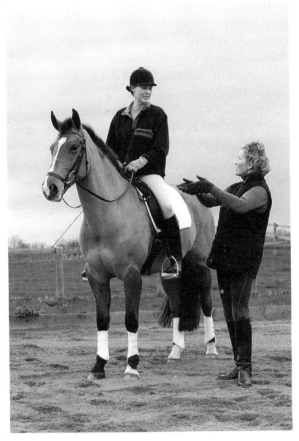

Fig. 1.1 The trainer must be a good communicator. (*Courtesy:* Elizabeth Furth)

pupils and establish the current state of affairs and evaluate how this may inhibit or enhance their performance.

It is not easy to 'read' people and the trainer can, on occasion, misread the signs. Sometimes the pupil may unwittingly give out confusing or misleading signs that we have to unravel.

Open mindedness

Trainers must be open to new ideas, both in the way that they teach and in the ways in which horse and rider learn.

Being yourself

Trainers must be themselves and develop their own philosophy, technique and characteristics. This is encompassed by 'image', for example the way we dress says a lot about who we are. Clearly the trainer must be encouraged to dress appropriately for the type of training being given, the weather and the circumstances. For example, when giving a lecture demonstration, team training, instructing in a riding school or a private yard, each will demand some modifications to the 'norm' – whatever that might be.

What other aspects should be considered when training the trainer? Potential or developing trainers must be encouraged to think about themselves as well as those they are about to train. They could perhaps perform a SWOT analysis to decide what their strengths, weaknesses, opportunities and threats are. This can cover a wide range of issues, for example:

- Strengths – enthusiasm, gift for communication.
- Weaknesses – lack of planning, lack of self discipline when planning own schedule and pricing structure.
- Opportunities – develop local Pony Club, teach other aspiring instructors.
- Threats – competition from others, lack of self confidence.

Ideally the strengths and opportunities should outweigh the weaknesses and threats, but by identifying the negative aspects of one's personality one can go a long way to overcoming them. Arguably one of the riding instructor's weakest areas is a lack of structure and planning of activities. Thus, a very important aspect of training others is to encourage them to be more organized. This is a relatively simple task with one horse and rider. Imagine that the rider wants to qualify his/her horse for the winter novice dressage championship. This is defined as a long term goal, but within this would be smaller goals, which are identified by working backwards from the main goal. Short term goals would include a number of qualifying competitions, warm up competitions and practice competitions. By evaluating past and current performance the trainer and rider can work together to establish specific goals for each competition; these can then be carried down to each lesson.

Life is more difficult if you have a mixed group of horses and riders. For example, at a riding club rally the goal becomes much more difficult to identify. The teacher has to try to identify a common thread that can stretch the most able but be adapted for those with problems. It is important that the goal is agreed with the participants at the outset and that the goal can be modified if, after an initial assessment, the original aim appears to be either too ambitious or not fulfilling enough.

Having identified the goal the next task is to plan the lesson to fit in with the time and facilities available. We very often try to fit too much into one lesson, thus cutting down the time for quality achievement. This is particularly important when training for competition or examination just because it has been covered in a lesson does not mean that the pupil can reproduce the work at a satisfactory standard. Perhaps the weekly leisure rider would prefer to have greater variety with less quality – this all has to be considered and agreed between pupil and teacher.

Having implemented the plan it is important to allow adequate feedback time. This should be a two-way communication with every effort being made to make the lesson finish on an upward note.

Therefore your ideal lesson structure would be as follows:

- Evaluate current and past competence and achievement of pupils.
- Agree the goals for the future and the day.
- Plan the lesson.
- Assess the riders.
- Adapt the plan and goal if necessary.
- Implement the plan.
- Evaluate the lesson, gain feedback and plan future strategies.

If you are involved in a series of lessons then planning and goal setting are relatively easy and can be done in advance. It is more difficult in a 'one-off' situation and often involves the trainer 'thinking on his/her feet'. However, if planning has become the norm then arriving at a swift decision based on discussion and ridden assessment becomes much easier.

In ideal training sessions the reward should be shared by all involved: the teacher, the pupil and the horse. If a session has not gone well, try to identify what went wrong – could it have been avoided or were the circumstances beyond your control? There always has to be an answer but, equally, there is always encouragement to be found.

This book aims to show how to use the philosophy 'Accentuate the positive, eliminate the negative' in the day-to-day teaching of riders and instructors.

2 Trainers and Their Roles

There is much more to teaching than merely explaining or showing a person how to do something.

Terminology

Firstly, it is useful to examine what is meant by a teacher. There is a plethora of terms used to describe people who 'teach' others and they all tend to have slightly different meanings and connotations. What do these terms mean in the context of the horse industry?

Coach
A coach is defined as a person who trains athletes or sports teams or as a private tutor employed to prepare a student for an examination. Equine teachers are rarely referred to as coaches, and perhaps the closest example is when teams of riders undertake intensive team training prior to a major international competition.

Trainer
A trainer is a person who makes others proficient with specialized instruction or practice, someone who trains either people or horses for specialized sporting events. This fits both our concept of the racehorse trainer who trains horses and the dressage trainer who works on both horse and rider.

Instructor
An instructor is a teacher who educates and provides knowledge, a person who gives a lesson.

Teacher
A teacher gives systematic instruction to help develop knowledge or

skill. In riding, an instructor or teacher is the commonly used term for those who teach people to ride.

Lecturer

A lecturer is a teacher in a college or university who teaches by formal discussion of a subject. In many cases the riding instructor also acts as a lecturer when teaching theoretical aspects of riding, teaching and stable management.

The riding teacher

Traditionally we have accepted that we learn from an authoritative teacher; experts impart their knowledge to those without it for the good of the pupil and we have accepted that, being older and wiser, the teacher knows what is good for the pupil. Providing that pupils accept that learning is necessary and desirable, they will learn by listening, taking in, remembering and acting in the way they have been taught.

Over the last 20 years the traditional hierarchy of teaching has been questioned. It is no longer thought that people should learn without questioning. Expertise is essential but should not create an elite with a group of dependants. These days pupils are encouraged to take responsibility for their own learning and part of the teaching process involves providing the skills needed to do this.

In educational terms this has led to a change from curriculum-led teaching to student-centred learning. The role of the teacher is to make learning easier by inspiring, advising and helping the learner. The decisions about what to learn, how to learn it and when to learn it, along with the responsibility for doing the learning, rest with the pupil. This fits in very well with the recognized role of the riding coach, but may not seem as applicable to teaching the class ride in the riding school. The times when we used to say 'Do as I say and don't ask questions' are over. In fact, whenever teaching, especially with new pupils or unfamiliar exercises, explanations as to why the aids are as they are or why an exercise is appropriate should be automatic.

Do I or can I act as an:

- *instructor* – directing activities and practices;
- *teacher* – imparting new knowledge, skills and ideas;
- *trainer* – improving skills and fitness;
- *motivator* – generating a positive and decisive approach;
- *disciplinarian* – determining a system of rewards and punishments;

- *manager and administrator* – organizing and planning, dealing with paperwork;
- *publicity agent* – controlling the public accolade;
- *social worker* – counselling and advising;
- *friend* – supporting and sustaining;
- *scientist* – analysing, evaluating and problem solving;
- *student* – willing to listen and learn, to think for myself and seek out new information;
- *guardian* – protecting from harm, injury and unhelpful influences.

Many of us have acted in all these roles at one time or another. It is worth studying each in more detail:

- An instructor is someone who directs activities and practices; in this sense it is the role of the Chief Instructor, in other words the person who organizes and supervises other teachers.
- The teacher imparts new knowledge, skills and ideas and is a role that most of us assume frequently. It is perhaps the aspect of our job that we enjoy the most, seeing horses and riders progress with our help.
- The trainer is defined here as the person who improves a rider's skills and fitness, in other words their role leads on from that of the teacher to help riders achieve their potential.

All these roles require you to be a motivator. Successful instructors/teachers/trainers generate a positive and decisive approach from their pupils. In order to be a motivator the trainer must have credibility and look the part (Fig. 2.1)

- Telling you that you have to be a disciplinarian sounds old fashioned and rather terrifying, but effective learning requires discipline from the pupil as well as motivation. You will work out your own system of rewards for your pupils depending on their age, ability and goals.
- The mere fact of living seems to generate paperwork. Organizing and planning and dealing with paperwork demands that you act as a manager and administrator. For example, if you are self-employed this may consist of handling your invoices and accounts, or it may be helping your pupils enter for examinations and competitions.
- When it all comes together and one of your pupils excels and

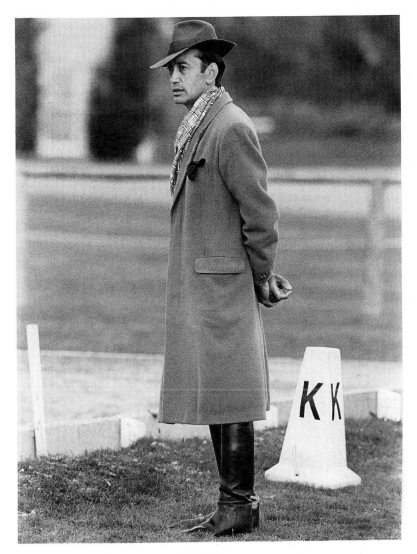

Fig. 2.1 The trainer should look the part. (*Courtesy:* Elizabeth Furth)

comes into the public eye, it will be up to you to act as 'publicity agent' to help him/her cope.

● Leading on from this, the teacher may have to act as guardian, protecting from harm, injury and unhelpful influences (Fig. 2.2).

● One of the most underestimated roles of the successful teacher is that of a social worker. Young people particularly will look to you for advice and much of the discussion that you have in the face of disappointment is, in effect, counselling (Fig. 2.3).

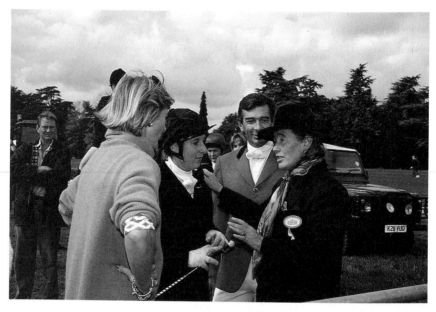

Fig. 2.2 The teacher may have to act as a guardian. (*Courtesy:* Elizabeth Furth)

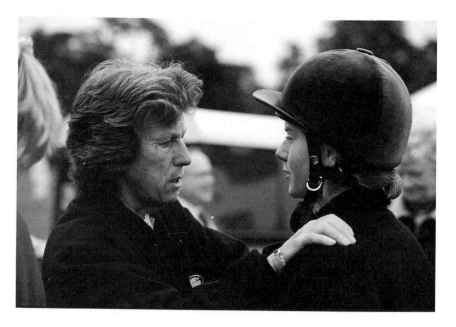

Fig. 2.3 Young riders may need their teacher to act as a counsellor. (*Courtesy:* Elizabeth Furth)

- As the relationship between pupil and trainer develops it is likely that the pupil will also turn to the trainer for support. This is different from counselling in that the pupil may be seeking non-judgemental friendship rather than advice.
- You may not have been good at science at school, but teaching riders and horses involves 'scientific' qualities such as analysing and evaluating performance and solving any problems that arise. All these tasks require discipline, consistency and concentration.
- None of us knows everything; indeed, as you learn more it becomes increasingly apparent just how much more there is to learn. The teacher must be willing to listen and learn, to think independently and to seek out new information.

As you can see there is a lot more to being a good riding teacher than horsemanship!

Qualities of a good riding teacher

A good riding teacher has:

- to inspire students to want to learn and achieve. Students who are motivated learn better. Motivation may be in the form of targets of achievement, for example passing an examination or being successful in a competition;
- ability to plan and organize teaching and training. Structured training gives a logical base to work from and enables the teacher to make the most of any learning situation;
- ability to demonstrate and explain the skill involved. For leaders to be credible their demonstrations should be effective. They should also be able to explain why a skill should be achieved to ensure that the pupil understands the validity of the exercise;
- ability to give understanding and knowledge in addition to skills. An appreciation of the structure of the horse, the way he moves and the demands of competition enables the student to understand the aids and movements more fully. An insight into the history of equitation helps students understand how training methods have been built up over the years;
- ability to see and correct errors in pupils and their horses. A good teacher must be able to correct riders' and horses' faults quickly and accurately. The teacher must be able to weigh up the relative

importance of the faults and assess how they relate to the horse's way of going;

- a pleasant, well-modulated voice. The voice must carry but not irritate or grate on the student;
- ability to communicate with and know students, to decide whether they need encouragement or to be driven with a certain amount of determination. Good teachers encourage students to talk, while they listen, and then put forward their own beliefs;
- ability to establish rapport with people;
- ability to overcome resistance to change;
- ability to react to many different and unexpected situations.

Above all, the riding teacher must be positive and build on the good to overcome weakness. A happy pupil is a learning pupil and remember to vary the technique to keep up the interest.

Establishing rapport

What does establishing rapport mean? It involves building trust and creating affinity between the teacher and the pupil. How do we go about this? The teacher must ensure that pupils feel confident to place themselves and their horses in the teacher's care. The teacher must ensure that pupils progress towards their chosen goals following an agreed timescale. This means that, as the teacher, you must have sufficient knowledge and credibility to feel confident that you can meet the needs of your client. This demands instructor qualifications or a strong background of equine expertise with an ability to communicate effectively.

All instructors must try and place themselves in the pupil's place, be it a child, a nervous adult or an ambitious competition rider. Only by trying to identify yourself with the pupil's needs and thoughts can you establish an affinity. This is one of the reasons why it can be difficult for a younger person to coach someone considerably older, as clearly you cannot know how it feels to be something you have never been! So, how else can the instructor tackle this? Talk to your clients and try to find out what makes them tick. If they have fears or self doubts, use your equine experience and try to allay them using reasoned discussion and suitable exercises.

We have already said that a happy pupil is a learning pupil and, usually, a learning pupil is a successful pupil, so make every effort to keep your pupil happy.

In the riding school situation it is very easy for the teacher to become bored and therefore disinterested. Compare this with the aerobics teacher at your local evening class who positively bubbles with enthusiasm. Try and focus on every lesson being rewarding for yourself and stimulating to the pupil. If you can finish with the participants still keen to carry on, you are on the winning path.

Encourage both the school and the participants to keep 'records of achievement'. For example:

Name: Emily   Class: Housewives' weekly class
Date: 18 May 1995
Today I managed to keep 'Toby' in canter all the way round the school.

It is very much easier to create rapport with individual riders, especially private clients with their own horses, who are all too often like hypochondriac patients who ring the doctor at every available moment to discuss the symptoms and treatments of their varying conditions! To keep a happy balance between clients feeling that you are pleased to work with them, and each feeling that they are your only client and demanding all your attention, can be quite tricky. Above all, always try to be honest with your pupils, not only in terms of your evaluation of their and their horses' abilities and aspirations, but also be honest with yourself.

- Have you given value for money?
- Have you sacrificed your principles?
- Are you, as the teacher, satisfied with the outcome of the lesson?
- Have you made every effort to satisfy the needs of the pupil?

Always give your clients the chance to talk about their needs, encourage them to see others teach and to experience other methods of teaching. Trust yourself to be able to deliver the goods, so that you are not afraid of competition. Remember, always be realistic and do not be dogmatic – many roads lead to Rome.

Overcoming resistance to change
This can be broken down into two main categories:

- the competition rider who has always worked along one system, for example he/she has always sat in the saddle on the approach to

show jumps and the trainer wishes the rider to adopt a light seat
for show jumping;
- the instructor who has always taught with no preconceived plan or
thoughts that all pupils are different.

One tool available to us is persuasion, but how can we use that tool?
Firstly, establish by questioning why the person uses their current
method. The rider might rely, for example, on sitting in the saddle in
order to keep the horse together. This will then give you the opportunity to discuss alternative methods; in fact, across country or racing
it is possible to keep the horse together from a light seat. To prove
your point use a demonstration, either ride the horse yourself or get
the pupil to try it out. Explain your reasons for wishing to change the
rider's technique – it is of course vital that the trainer has all the facts
at his/her fingertips – and brings forward examples to illustrate the
argument. Change should never be made for the sake of change but
because there are valid reasons to make that change. Perhaps in this
case the rider is inclined to 'fire' the horse at the fences and it is not so
easy to do this from a light seat which gives a valid reason to try and
implement change.

The resistance to change may be stronger in the second example.
The concept of student-centred learning is still not widely accepted by
the riding teacher or pupils, but there is no doubt that when students
have to accept some responsibility for learning then their understanding and feel is better based, although pupils may feel that they
would have benefited from being constantly corrected by the
instructor. When the instructor has taken all the responsibility for the
student's learning, the quieter and more introvert pupils in the ride
often have gaps in their knowledge and feel, because they are too shy
to ask for clarification of points they do not understand. On the other
hand, extrovert pupils can 'kid' the instructor that they know it all
unless they are asked specific questions or involved in specific exercises to help identify the gaps in their knowledge. These reasons need
to be discussed with instructors to help persuade those that are
reluctant to change their teaching methods. Indeed the word 'adapt' is
probably better than 'change' as it does not sound so radical.

Instructors are often resistant to change because they feel that they
are already being successful, they use the argument 'well, all my pupils
pass their BHS Stage II first time'. Just as when Great Britain was
winning all the medals for eventing, it was said 'why should we train,
we win medals anyway?'. Several years later there was surprise and

consternation when we stopped winning. Success depends on having a strong base and training now takes place on a national basis. We have to try and convince the teacher that success on its own is not a strong enough measure.

We seem to have an inherent resistance to change, perhaps it is laziness that makes us all guilty of thinking that if it works why change it, rather than trying it and seeing if it is better. Certainly change for its own sake is poor policy, but growth within oneself can benefit all concerned, and as we grow we need to adapt and adjust. The expectations of people change, especially young people. The successful teacher must be ready to meet these new expectations and if this necessitates change in our own teaching methodology or communication skills, so be it.

Unpredictability of horses

The riding teacher's biggest problem is that horses are very unpredictable and the instructor must be able to react to many different and unexpected situations. The unexpected is less likely to occur in a riding school because most of the horses have met the various situations before, but riding school horses have to be made, few are born that way. It is recommended that the horses are introduced into their schoolmaster role by the more experienced riders and are only gradually introduced to the more novice riders.

If you are teaching people on their own horses at the Pony Club or riding club and a horse or pony behaves out of character, try to ascertain why:

- Is the horse underexercised and overfed? – a management problem.
- Is the horse in pain? – horses invariably run away from physical pain and some may rear, buck or nap. In some cases horses will misbehave in anticipation of pain or fear which could be caused, for example, by bad riding, overfacing the horse or unjust punishment.
- Is the rider nervous, lacking in confidence or frightened?

The action to be taken by the instructor will vary according to the particular problem, but in all cases the most important action must be to try and ensure the safety of the rider. You may have to:

- stop the exercise completely;
- ride the horse yourself to evaluate the problem more thoroughly;
- modify the exercise;
- get extra, experienced help if it is available.

Accidents

No matter how careful an instructor is there will always be times when the rider or the horse and rider have a fall. In these days when litigation is becoming the norm, the instructor needs to take great care how this situation is handled. The circumstances of course vary depending on whether it is a riding school, club or a private client taught by a freelance instructor. All instructors should have an insurance policy that covers them for public liability. It is also highly recommended that all instructors have a current first aid certificate. Regardless of how simple a fall appears to be, all commercial riding schools and clubs are required to record the fall and its nature in a book or on a report form. The report should include date, time, place, name of pupil, name of instructor and qualifications if appropriate and a simple description of what happened and the action taken. The report should be signed by the pupil, instructor and, if possible, a witness. If the accident is of a serious nature, for example, concussion, a broken limb or severe cuts and bruising so that the pupil is unable to carry on, the instructor must make sure that the record is accurate and complete, including perhaps a sketch. Freelance instructors would be well advised to maintain a similar record; a client may not go to their solicitor for a long time after an accident and it may be years before the case gets into court, and memories fade.

Mercifully most falls, whilst being 'an h'awful thing' in the words of Jorrocks, are not so serious that the rider suffers more than a blow to his/her pride. There are some guidelines to follow even if the fall does not appear serious:

- Ask the rider if he/she is hurt. If the answer is 'no', then allow the rider to remount and continue the lesson. Be vigilant and if in any doubt, suggest that the rider calls it a day.
- Never allow a rider who has previously lost consciousness, even momentarily, to remount. Any blow to the head needs to be treated with great care; the rider may feel fine at the time but can become dizzy later, and the delay can be as much as 24 hours.

- Some riders are very brave and want to continue regardless. However, if you are in any doubt, the onus is on you as the instructor to say 'no'.
- When there is a serious accident, the lesson will have to be stopped immediately and help summoned along with the emergency services.

The Reporting of Injuries, Diseases and Dangerous Occurrences Regulations (RIDDOR) 1985 require employers, people in control of premises and, in some cases, the self-employed to report certain types of injury, occupational ill health and dangerous occurrences, to their enforcing authority. In the case of riding establishments the enforcing authority is the local environmental health department. If someone dies, suffers one of the following injuries or if there is a dangerous occurrence, the employer must notify the authority immediately, normally by phone, and send a written report within seven days:

- fracture of the skull, spine or pelvis;
- fracture of any bone in the arm or leg (not hand or foot);
- loss of a hand, foot, finger, thumb or toe;
- loss of sight of an eye or a penetrating injury to the eye;
- electric shock needing immediate medical treatment or resulting in loss of consciousness;
- loss of consciousness resulting from lack of oxygen;
- illness requiring treatment caused by inhalation, ingestion or absorption through the skin of any substance;
- illness requiring treatment caused by exposure to a pathogen or infected material;
- any other injury that results in hospitalization for more than 24 hours.

The authority must also be notified if employees are off work or cannot carry out their normal duties for more than three consecutive days as a result of an accident at work.

First aid

You should always know where the first aid facilities are. Indeed freelance teachers may find it useful to carry their own first aid kit containing:

- crepe and adhesive bandages;
- cottonwool;
- individually wrapped plasters;
- antiseptic solution;
- non-adherent dressings, e.g. Melonin;
- safety pins;
- scissors;
- disposable gloves.

Treatment of injury

It is advised that all teachers attend a recognized first aid course, and this is essential for membership of the BHS Register of Instructors. Small cuts and grazes should be dealt with calmly and correctly. The first thing to do is to assess the severity of the wound and decide if medical help is needed. In cases of more severe injury, emergency procedures should be followed and help summoned as soon as possible.

Health and safety

The teacher has a responsibility for the health and safety of the pupils during the lesson. You must adhere to the following guidelines to avoid being held responsible for any accidents. It will also reinforce safety to the pupils.

Before the lesson:

- check that equipment, horses, machinery and the location are all as safe as practicable;
- check that regulations and codes of practice are adhered to;
- make sure the teaching method is free from unnecessary risks;
- wear the necessary protective clothing and insist that pupils do also;
- check that pupils have no physical defect that may put them at risk.

During the lesson:

- stress all the safety points;
- explain safety regulations;
- ensure safe methods are used;
- point out known risks and hazards and show how they may be avoided.

Riding is a high risk sport and it is part of the teacher's job to use commonsense and to take specific precautions where appropriate. No matter how safety-conscious a teacher may be, accidents will happen and the teacher must know the steps to be followed should this occur.

One way to minimize the risks is to be aware of them in the first place. This means that the teacher must have an indepth knowledge of horses and how they are likely to react in different circumstances. This will allow the teacher to ensure that practices and situations promote safe conditions for the riders. Appropriate rules, such as the rules of the school, should be enforced and the potential dangers and hazards of being with horses appreciated. All riders should be made aware of any health and safety guidelines that are in operation.

Insurance is essential for both teachers and riders and should cover both public liability and personal accident. Options for the self-employed include private medical treatment and hospitalization insurance.

Your responsibilities

Facilities
Not all places where riding or stable management instruction take place are purpose-built; many are converted buildings which are not ideal. If the place where you teach is using horses for hire or reward, ensure that the establishment is licensed to do so by the local authority and preferably a governing body such as the BHS. Make it your practice to check out the current health and safety regulations covering the establishment and always make sure that you and your pupils are aware of basic emergency procedures in the case of an accident.

Equipment
The horses, tack and any other equipment used must be suitable for

the task in hand. If anything is in need of repair or maintenance then report it to the relevant person. Never modify equipment; it may make it potentially hazardous – even putting a twist in a stirrup leather could be perceived as a modification. Make sure that the equipment is the correct size for the rider, for example, adult-length reins are too long for children and they could catch their foot in the resulting loop. Keep both size and age in mind when selecting the horse, pony or equipment to be used. Ensure that equipment is put away safely, for example, jump poles and wings piled in the corner of the school can constitute a hazard. Particularly with beginner riders and children, be prepared to take the time to explain how to use any equipment safely.

Communication

Communication with the emergency services is essential. Unless you have a mobile phone it may be sensible to refuse to teach if a phone is not available. In addition there should be a list of contact names, addresses and phone numbers positioned near the phone in case of an emergency.

General guidelines for safe teaching

Preparation

- Explain the day-to-day safety code of conduct.
- As far as possible eliminate potential hazards.
- Check pupils' previous knowledge and experience.
- Explain the safety and emergency procedures.
- Plan and organize to allow sufficient space.
- Take time to explain the use of equipment, etc. to new riders and children.

Injury

- Do not diagnose and treat any but the most superficial injury.
- Keep calm and prevent others losing their calm or interfering.
- If in doubt do nothing until qualified help arrives.
- Offer comfort and reassurance whilst ensuring the safety of others.
- In the event of serious accident try to remember exactly what happened, when and how.
- Complete an accident report form.

Warm up and cool down

● Both horse and rider require adequate warm up and cool down periods to prevent injury.

Dress

● Insist on correct headwear and footwear.
● Dress may be casual or formal but must be appropriate and safe.
● Spectacles should contain plastic lenses.

In order to stay safe you may have to err on the side of caution. Some riders are very brave, perhaps braver than their ability level. Do not be tempted to let pupils be overbold or to ride on through injury – they may frighten themselves or have an accident.

3 Pupils and Their Goals

Where does one start when coaching competitors? One of the main criteria is to persuade competitors to believe in themselves and their horses. The blend of temperament of horse and rider is also very important, for example, not everybody is designed to work with stallions. Mares can be particularly delicate in their temperament and like to establish partnerships, rather than follow orders.

The first question that any trainer needs to ask when helping a rider to set goals is, 'Why does this person want to learn?'. There are probably a variety of reasons and in order for the teacher to ascertain the best method and approach for a particular rider, the reason why he/she has embarked on one or more lessons needs to be established.

At one level it may be simply that the customer is, say, a young man with a horse-riding girlfriend who wants to go with her on a trekking holiday so he decides to take some lessons so that he can create a reasonably good impression. This means that the long term goal is for the rider to be competent in walk, trot and canter. To enable him to impress his girlfriend he must be sufficiently confident and familiar with the procedures so that the whole thing seems natural. The teacher must break down the long term goal into achievable chunks, taking into account the time and funds available. In this case the finer points of rider position are relatively unimportant. The key factors are:

- safety;
- security;
- sufficient knowledge to give confidence.

Another example may be the businessman who has contacts who hunt and feels that he would like to join them. He has a little experience but lacks confidence in his ability to keep up with the Field in a country that demands the ability to gallop and jump. The client would perceive it as cowardly were he not able to jump with the rest of the Field, so he

24

needs to feel confident to jump, stay in control and enjoy the social aspects of a day's hunting. The last point may not concern us, but by achieving the first two we can make the third a feasible proposition. As with the first scenario, the niceties of position have to be weighed up against the effectiveness of the aids. Sometimes these two are hard to separate because the position often influences the effectiveness of the aids; this is a very important point to validate with your pupil – he must be convinced that there is a good reason for the teacher concentrating on his position (Fig. 3.1), as he would probably much rather be learning to jump immediately! Again, the long term goal of being able to hunt up with the Field, jumping with the others, needs to be broken down into smaller goals.

It is essential that clients always feel that they have achieved the goal of the lesson and, if for some reason, they have not, the teacher must be able to talk it through with them. Perhaps there were factors affecting the lesson which were not conducive to learning, for example, the weather or the timing, or at the end of the day the client may be physically and mentally tired. Maybe on this occasion the horse had not given of his best. If clients are being taught on their own horses, the teacher needs to be very tactful in any criticism of the horses. Owners are usually fond of their animals and may resent such

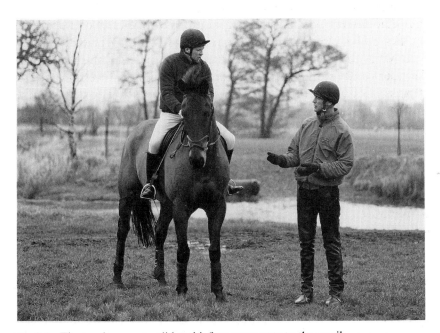

Fig. 3.1 The teacher must validate his/her comments to the pupil.

criticism, even if the teacher knows that they are the wrong vehicles for continuing success.

Goal setting is difficult when riders are not setting the goal but having it set for them by another person, often a parent. In this situation the teacher needs to be very strong; the parent's goal and the achievable goal may be poles apart, and it needs considerable tact to guide the parent in the right direction. The parent has to be persuaded to accept smaller goals in order to build up to the ultimate goal. For example, a parent may want his/her child to compete in the European pony dressage team championships. The child is 13 years old with an obedient but moderately-moving pony. What can the instructor do? First of all, evaluate the qualities needed to get into the team and then decide if the child has the necessary credentials. First and foremost, has the child the time and the inclination to commit himself/herself to the discipline involved – how single-minded is the child? Even if the pony is lacking talent, if the rider is committed enough some progress may be made. However, a suitable starting point has to be identified, be it a Pony Club competition or a winter unaffiliated competition. Even on the way to this, small goals need to be set and agreed with the parent, and the outcomes of each goal discussed with all the participating parties.

What other sorts of riders are there? There is the person who simply rides for social and physical recreation, whose needs are just as important as those of our would-be international rider. Often the rider with less ambition is more difficult to satisfy than the more ambitious rider. Try and ascertain at the start of either a series of lessons or at the beginning of a single lesson what the rider would like to achieve. The answer may be 'I would like to canter better'; we then have to define what the rider means by that by asking a series of questions:

'I want to bump less in the saddle.'
'On a scale of one to ten, how would you define your "bumping"?'
'Five out of ten'.

The instructor's task is then to get the rider to feel that he/she is bumping less and can evaluate this by working up the scale to a perfect ten. It is not the purpose of this book to tell you how to do this – you have various options open, and the success of the exercise you choose is based on the response from your client. Not all clients will respond in the same way to the same exercise. Clearly you need to achieve six out of ten, and hopefully start at that level at the beginning of the next lesson, depending on the time the rider has available for practice. The most important thing is that clients feel that they have achieved something during the lesson. On the subject of achievement, remember that most people respond better to praise than constant criticism. This does not mean that you cannot correct them, but simply that you should recognize achievement, however small.

The next category of rider to consider is the career student, that is the person who feels that he/she wishes to either ride or teach as a means of earning a living. Let us consider first the person who wishes to become a professional teacher; clearly, having a defined structure to follow makes long-term strategies relatively simple. However, each person's idea of 'long term' may vary, and few set out intending to become Fellows of the British Horse Society while many wish to become Assistant Instructors.

Goal setting for the career student may start at a very early stage, for example when making the decision at school which subjects to take at GCSE. The next goals may be set when he or she enrols at college or starts at a riding school. The college course may last one or more academic years with clear goals, such as examinations, each term. The riding school or training centre may have courses from three to twelve months in duration with goals set at strategic points. Where funding is available these goals may be of paramount importance, but as we have already outlined, goal setting is a key component of all good teaching.

For most instructors the greatest rewards come from teaching successful people, but great care must be taken that instructors do not impose too high a target for their pupils. Some encouragement and leadership is often needed but, equally, realism regarding the talents of both horse and rider is essential.

For example, you may have a horse and rider qualified for Badminton but when they get there are they going to be able to cope, especially with the cross country? No-one can say with certainty, but the rider's experience will give you a fairly good idea. If you do decide to go, what are you hoping to achieve – to get round and complete the event or to win, to come in the top half, or to get in the prize money? Setting a suitable target can make all the difference. The stress imposed on a rider trying to win is probably only equalled by the stress of being a first-time Badminton rider. Evaluate how the horse and rider cope with stress and take suitable action.

The reason for goal setting is to create a feeling that the participants are always the 'winners'. If riders do not perceive themselves as having 'won' then the instructor must give them and the others involved a clear reason why a 'win' has not been achieved on this particular occasion. Above all, pupils should enjoy themselves (Fig. 3.2). There will always be people who want to achieve at all costs and have the 'killer instinct'; they are usually the top-class competitors. Such riders need to have equally aggressive trainers who are cool and objective. These qualities are not easily found and they tend to be inherent in the person, rather than taught. However, there are people who have the 'killer instinct' and are not aware of it. Sometimes a particular occurrence triggers their awareness, such as a slightly insulting or condescending remark by another. The trainer may be able to uncover this special hidden feeling in discussion of why the 'win situation' has not come about.

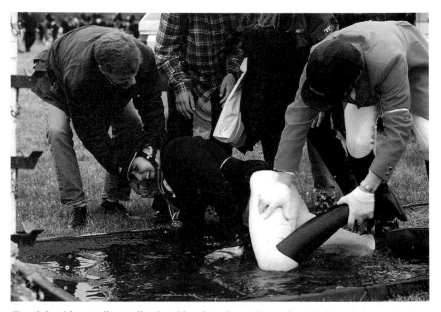

Fig. 3.2 Above all, pupils should enjoy themselves, though I would not suggest ducking every pupil in the water jump! (*Courtesy:* Elizabeth Furth)

Now let us examine some examples which may be found in a practical situation.

Example one

Danny is a 24-year-old man with no riding experience, whose long term goal is to accompany his girlfriend on a trekking holiday in

Scotland. It is now October and the holiday is next summer so the instructor has ten months to help prepare Danny. He rides on average once a week which will give in the region of 35 lessons. The first thing to do is to set medium and short term goals. It is easiest to do this by working backwards; Danny should be hacking out by lesson 25 which means that he will have to be cantering in company, outdoors, by lesson 20.

Thus lessons 20 to 25 must include walk, trot and canter, and learning the codes for riding out in groups. Lessons 15 to 20 should be outside in an enclosed field, building confidence and practising skills. Lessons 10 to 15 should be riding in a group in a manege or school, practising walk, trot and canter. Lessons 5 to 10 should be learning the basic skills for starting and stopping, as an individual initially and then progressing to riding in a group. Lessons 1 to 5 should establish confidence and position, teach the basic aids, get the riding muscles fit and allow the rider to begin to understand the horse.

Each lesson should be planned to have its own short term goal. For example, in lesson 1 Danny will learn to mount and dismount, walk, halt and do a few steps in sitting trot. While these may seem very simple goals to us, they demand quite complex co-ordinated reactions from a beginner rider. Try to remember when you last learned a new skill, and how difficult it was to master.

Example two

Carol is a 25-year-old woman whose long term goal is to compete at Osberton three day event and to finish in the top half. Osberton is in September and the horse, which is Intermediate with 23 points, all gained with its present owner, is coming back into work in January. Carol has competed at one-day level in Novice and Intermediate events with this horse, but she has another job and is an amateur competitor. Carol must qualify to compete at Osberton by completing the necessary number of competitions with clear rounds cross country. Again it is useful to work backwards; her last competition will be two weeks before Osberton, i.e. the end of August. How many times will she compete prior to Osberton? This could amount to ten events, based on running every two weeks on average. Individual goals should be set for each competition, depending on Carol's performance in previous competitions.

Carol will have one lesson a week from February until Osberton.

She will enter extra dressage and show jumping competitions as necessary to refine these disciplines, and individual goals will be set for these. The goal at a dressage competition must be always that the horse and rider, especially the horse, perform to the best of their current ability. Dressage sheets can then be evaluated and where a consistent problem is identified, for example, the halts are not straight and square, this can be worked on until the marks reflect an improvement. The goal is set – to improve the halt – and then achieved.

The general show jumping goal at every competition should be that the rider is never caught unawares through lack of attention to detail. This includes walking the course, noting times, checking the going, walking the distances and noticing any distracting activity that may affect the horse. There may be specific goals such as the horse needs to learn to become more agile and adjust the length of his stride because he always tends to make up too much ground in the combination. Trainer and rider will also work on this problem at home, setting smaller goals within each lesson. For example, the trainer could start with a double at 21 ft (6.5 m) wide and 3 ft 7 in (1.10 m) high, the approach is in canter with a placing pole 18 ft (5.5 m) in front of the first element. When the horse successfully negotiates this exercise in good balance and rhythm he has achieved a mini-goal and can move on.

You may be thinking 'Well, I do all that anyway' – good, just reflect on your goals and lesson structure and refine them as necessary. Remember the following points at each lesson:

- Negotiate the goal.
- Build confidence.
- Establish rapport.
- Build respect.
- Raise awareness of pupils to their own and the horse's reactions.
- Always finish on a positive note.
- Outline the likely goal for the next lesson.

In many cases riders will have problems that need to be sorted out. In order to help riders solve problems it is first necessary for them to trust their trainer so that the trainer can help them explore the perceived problem so that both parties know what they are dealing with. Why is the rider frightened to get on that particular horse? Why has the horse started to refuse to jump? Once the problem has been identified trainer and rider have to come to a decision that is mutually acceptable and then act on the basis of that decision.

This process is divided into three stages:

● the building relationship;
● exploring and clarifying the problem;
● planning for action.

Remember that your pupil will be expecting you, as the teacher and expert, to take control and responsibility for the lesson, while you want the pupil to start to take responsibility for his/her own learning. At first the pupil may find this disconcerting and it is important that the concept of student-centred learning is introduced in such a way that the pupil does not feel that the teacher is 'opting out' and letting the pupil do all the work. The idea is to build a relationship where the pupil does not feel inadequate or inferior; it is easy to intimidate the less experienced or nervous rider. Pupils can then be encouraged to take control of their own learning by assessing themselves, knowing when and how to ask for help and deciding what steps to follow.

Most competition riders are familiar with student-centred learning; they have clearly identifiable goals and how these goals are met is negotiated between the pupil and the trainer. Conversely, with a group of novice riders it is often better that the teacher sets out the lesson and its objectives and in addition the proposed sequence of lessons which follow. This does not mean, however, that the pupils cannot be encouraged to assess themselves, and be educated to know when and how to ask for help.

Your aim as a riding teacher is to produce someone who can ride just as well when you are not there as when you are present. The rider should not become dependent on the presence of the teacher in order to produce the desired work.

Building the relationship

Respect
The trainer must have respect for the pupil's ability to learn and accept that you are equal in ability overall. In this situation you have skills that the other does not. It can be difficult to keep this in mind, especially when teaching children or people with learning difficulties and it is possible to make them feel 'stupid'. Always look for the good points and utilize the pupil's different way of perceiving the world.

Empathy

The trainer must remember what it is like to be a pupil and pick up and understand the pupil's feelings. This is difficult if, for example, you are dealing with a nervous rider and you have never felt any fear of horses. Put yourself back at school and try to remember what it is like to be learning something new and when everybody else catches on more quickly than you. Or the teacher uses words you cannot understand. Or you do not get on with the rest of the group. Or you find what you are learning so difficult that you cannot enjoy it. Or you have just achieved something you found very difficult and you did not receive any praise.

Genuineness

Be yourself, relate to your pupil on a person-to-person basis by sharing experiences where appropriate – explain that you too found this difficult at first. Be human, have a joke with the pupil, or discipline them as necessary.

Exploring and clarifying the problem

Try to get pupils to identify their own weaknesses and to find their own sources of help by using the skills of questioning, paraphrasing, summarizing and confronting the pupils. The following questions may help:

- What is the most difficult part?
- What do you think?
- What makes you think that...?
- How did you do that?
- What would happen if...?
- So the most important aspects are...?
- What have you just done?
- How does that compare with the instructions?
- Last time you said..., but now you....

Planning for action

Pupils must be encouraged to assess their progress, their aims and how to achieve them. This is done by:

(1)   evaluating – what worked best?
        – what was good/bad?
(2)   problem solving – what might happen if. . .?
        – how will you feel if. . .?
        – what information do you need first?
(3)   objective setting – what do you wish to practise most?
        – when do you plan to start/finish?

Just as people have different learning styles so teachers and coaches have different styles and methods. The really great coach/pupil partnerships are often due to the complementary nature of their inherent talents; look at the success of the Ginny Elliot team. However there are certain qualities that a good riding teacher should aim to develop.

Encouraging pupils to be positive

Encouraging pupils to be positive is a key factor in successful learning. Sometimes it is useful to ask students to use a range of marks to evaluate the depth of a problem and then to encourage improvement by building up the 'marks'. For example, if the teacher asks the pupil 'How do you feel the horse is going now?' and the pupil replies, 'I haven't got enough in my hand', the teacher should ask the pupil to quantify this by saying, 'On a scale of one to ten, how much have you got?'. The answer is 'Maybe five' so the teacher tackles the problem by saying, 'By either increasing the activity or by improving the rein contact, tell me when it has got to six'. This method may not suit all pupils or fit every circumstance, but it is a useful approach for riders who tend to have a slightly negative attitude.

Keeping a learning record

Keeping a learning record helps pupils to take control of their own learning; it enables them to analyse what has been learnt and to organize how and when to work. Exactly the same process can be used in the classroom when helping pupils organize project work or in the manege when planning a horse's schooling regime, or in the stable yard when organizing the stable management of a horse prior to a competition. Learning records are a relatively recent introduction and many pupils will find it hard to organize enough time to write them up.

The riding trainer may find it useful to encourage the pupil to use other forms of evidence such as video and memory.

Prompt questions on the content
What do you count as the most/least significant moments in this session?

What have you learnt from this session?

How did you feel about...?

Was there anything that did not work for you? Why do you think that was?

Have you had any feedback from anybody (colleagues, friends or teacher)?

4 The Learning Environment

Factors influencing learning

There are a large number of factors that can help or hinder learning. The four main factors are:

- goal
- learning environment
- personal characteristics
- learning process.

The goal
The job people hope to end up in or their aim in undertaking learning determines what they need to learn; the teacher will have helped them establish and define their long and short term goals. Whatever the goal the trainee must not be afraid to make mistakes – it is like training horses; if the horse does not make a mistake you can be sure that the rider has not asked a great deal of him. Mistakes are an important part of learning and remember that experimentation or doing is ultimately how we learn best.

The learning environment
Before designing a lesson plan that aims to teach a skill or achieve a short term goal, the riding teacher has to consider the learning environment which consists of three factors:

- the pupil
- the teacher
- the facilities.

The pupils' motivation to learn the skill will significantly affect how effectively learning takes place, as will their aptitude or talent.

Sometimes a highly motivated pupil will out-perform those with greater talent but less motivation. Motivated pupils are undoubtedly easier to teach! We have already outlined the qualities of a good riding teacher; the teacher's ability to teach effectively will also affect the learning outcomes. The facilities needed should be suitable for the identified goal; if the facilities are inadequate the goal will not be achieved. Remember that 'facilities' includes the time available as well as the horses, equipment and riding areas.

Personal characteristics
Each of the factors already mentioned is further influenced by personal characteristics such as:

- physical state, e.g. tiredness
- fitness
- mental state, e.g. anxiety
- age
- sex
- degree of maturity
- intelligence.

Each pupil is an individual and must be treated as such for the best results.

The learning process
The instructor is responsible for making the best use of what the pupil can offer in the way of physical and mental ability. Interesting and clear lessons will motivate the student and enhance progression, although the progress made may be physically limited by the speed at which the student can master the techniques. The instructor must bear in mind that some students are attempting to learn a skill up to only a modest level for their own enjoyment. A competent teacher is likely to be able to raise the ceiling on this pre-conceived level, but to prevent the teacher's own frustration and the pupils' misery it should be remembered that some pupils will not have the motivation to go as far as their aptitude would allow.

Trainees must have a good rapport with their trainers and not be put off or made to feel uncomfortable by other trainees. Adult novice riders often find learning difficult if they are in a ride with children. Personal factors such as learning style and study skills affect the learning process. Both may be affected by the past experiences of learning.

Fear, boredom and excitement

Fear, boredom and excitement can help or hinder learning and achievement. Different people with different personalities and different skills will find different things frightening, boring or exciting. We are afraid of doing things that may hurt us, physically or emotionally, and the fear may be due to lack of confidence or ability or previous bad experience. Exciting things stretch our ability, bringing with them an emotional or physical thrill. When we become used to doing something it becomes boring, it is no longer a challenge.

Table 4.1 Factors influencing learning.

• past experience of learning	• school may not have been a positive experience
• awareness of the learning process	• do pupils know what is involved?
• blockages to learning	• fear, pain, boredom
• personal learning style	• the character of the pupils
• learning skills	• do they pay attention and take in what you say?
• impact of colleagues	• competition may help or hinder learning depending on the pupils' characters
• impact of the trainer	• do you get on? do they respect you?
• methods of learning	• must be relevant
• climate	• the right atmosphere
• job content	• is the content of your teaching relevant?
• range of opportunities	• make it fun
• impact of shocks/mistakes	• getting a fright may be devastating to pupils
• recognition of need	• treat them as individuals

Facilitating learning

People learn best in a non-judgemental, non-threatening atmosphere and it is up to the teacher to create this atmosphere. In order for people to learn, the teacher must help pupils to:

- identify and deal with the various resistances to change that may result from learning;
- come to terms with personal strengths and weaknesses which may become apparent during learning;
- apply the new knowledge/skill to their real situation;
- plan for future learning.

This is a support role and involves counselling skills, in other words helpful behaviour that is easily understood by the pupil. The aim is to improve the pupil's self esteem and this is achieved by:

- establishing trust so that the pupil feels secure and sufficiently confident to reveal worries, fears and aspirations;
- being positive so that the pupil will share this positive attitude.

Bear in mind the following points:

- Counsel pupils individually and respect their need for privacy.
- Encourage pupils to express themselves.
- Achieve empathy by putting yourself in their place and reflecting their feelings.
- Be specific with encouragement.
- Find them interesting – develop your listening skills.
- Do not be over critical.
- Beware of reacting aggressively if the pupil is antagonistic – this may be a defence against feelings of inadequacy.
- Be positive and praise positive attitudes.

Teaching riding should be a client-centred process (Fig. 4.1) with the time taken to achieve goals being determined by the client. This will result in effective learning because the client does not feel threatened

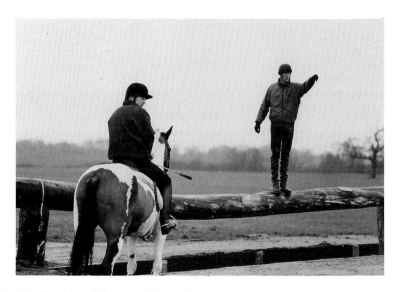

Fig. 4.1   Teaching riding should be a client-centred process.

and pressured. Traditionally the teacher has dictated how long it will take to teach a class of pupils a new skill or knowledge. This is didactic and can be highly threatening to less able or experienced pupils, resulting in less efficient learning.

Table 4.2   Facilitating learning – activities that enable pupils to learn more about horses.

Active activities (those the pupil does)

Creating
- Write an essay or notes
- Produce a project
- Give a talk
- Make a model
- Draw a picture, plan or diagram
- Take a photograph
- Make a film, video, tape or slides
- Write a short story that is well researched
- Any form of synthesis where something is built up or put together

Solving
- Objective test (test of facts)
- Practical test of problem solving
- Experiment to solve a problem
- Knowledge test
- Comprehension test
- Application test
- Buzz group (impromptu discussion on a specific topic)
- Judge a competition
- Place in order of merit
- Identification test
- Answer questions
- Literary search
- Evaluate information

Using
- Knowledge
- Practical practice (common in riding schools)
- Role play
- Discussion group
- Business games
- Practical competition
- Practical examination of competence
- Teaching aids, audio and/or visual
- Programmed learning
- Fill in handout
- Use teaching pack
- Demonstrate skill

Table 4.2 continued

Passive activities (those the pupil has done to him/her)

Indirect (may be instructor guided)
- Read a book, magazine, paper, map, wallchart or poster
- Watch and listen to a film, video, TV or slides
- Listen to radio, tape or record
- Smell various odours
- Feel shape and texture of various objects
- Visit show and study trade stands
- Visit sale, competition, display, demonstration or exhibition
- Enter environment, e.g. the Spanish Riding School in Vienna
- Be frightened by an experience

Direct (instructor based activities)
- A tour or walk
- A demonstration
- A led discussion
- Instructor answers questions
- Dictated or copied notes
- External reinforcement
- External motivation

Questioning

Talking and asking questions are our main methods of verbal communication. There are many uses of questions and the appropriateness of the questions is important. The reasons for asking them include:

- to get information – about something you don't know;
                            – to find out how much people know;
- to express disagreement;
- to make people be aware;
- to involve people;
- to put people on the spot.

How a question is asked, such as the phrasing, the underlying implications, the tone of voice and the likely effect of the question on the pupil, will alter its effectiveness. If you are questioning someone who has made a mistake, consider the effect on the person of these different questions:

- Why did you?
- Why didn't you?

● Did you know?
● What made you?

Always consider the aims of your questioning and decide whether the phrasing of the question allowed you to achieve your aims.

Developing questioning techniques
During a lesson you will ask questions to get the pupil thinking. It is important that questions are asked at the right time and in the right way.

When to ask questions

● during the introduction;
● when introducing information;
● during practice;
● when correcting errors;
● during the summary.

How to ask questions   The question may test key points and require a specific piece of information, such as where do the side reins attach? Other questions require more thought and demand explanation in the answer, for example, what are the possible safety hazards? Questions that start with what, where, when and how will usually receive an explanation and can be usefully followed with 'Why', to get a deeper explanation.

Who to ask the question of   If you want to ask a general or 'overhead' question, the quickest off the mark answers, but everyone has to think. Or you can overhead and nominate by asking the question, pausing and then giving the name of the person who should answer. This makes everybody think and stay involved, but allows the teacher to select who will answer. Or you can nominate by giving a name and then asking the question. This is useful if one pupil has specific knowledge or experience that you want the other pupils to hear.

It is common knowledge that if you want the right answer then you have to ask the right question. Questions have three main purposes:

● to test related knowledge;
● to identify reasoning ability;

- to help solve problems.

There are some simple guidelines that should always be kept in mind when questioning learners:

- Keep the question clear and simple.
- Use simple language which the pupil can understand.
- Avoid questions that test powers of expression.
- Avoid questions about the obvious.
- Do not ask trick questions.
- Avoid questions with yes or no answers.
- In an assessment situation, prepare the questions in advance.

Words mean different things to different people and questions and observations should be kept as simple as possible.

Take for example the teacher who is testing the related knowledge that a pupil has of the anatomy of the lower leg of the horse.

Question: 'Name and designate the tendons and ligaments below the knee'.

The pupil may not know what the word 'designate' means; the phraseology must be kept simple.

Question: 'Show me where the tendons and ligaments are and give me their names, if you can'.

This is a much more friendly approach and will still establish the relevant related knowledge.

Horsemanship is full of jargon and the use of simple language is of great importance, especially when teaching children or newcomers to the sport.

Use the words when, why and where to identify the reasoning ability of a pupil, especially for the purposes of evaluation, for example:

'When does your horse feel at its best?'

'Why do you find it is necessary to go into sitting trot to ride shoulder in?'

'Where are the tangent points on a circle?'

'How can the tangent points on a circle help you to ride a better shaped circle?'

Yes or no answers are rarely sufficiently expansive to give the whole answer; equally the pupil has a 50% chance of getting the answer right. For example, the question 'Did you put three strides between those two fences?' would be better phrased as 'How many strides did you feel that the horse put in between the two fences?'.

If you normally teach graduates and serious students who have progressed some way down their equine educational pathway you may be able to ask, 'Did you feel that the longitudinal bend was commensurate with the line of the circle?'. Reduced to simple language the question becomes, 'Did you feel that your pony's body was following the line of the circle?'. The standard of the question is still quite demanding in terms of the need for knowledge and feel from the rider, but it is expressed in a more simplistic way. The question could be broken down further:

Question: 'Was your pony following the line of the circle?'
Answer: 'I don't know.'
Question: 'Is his nose following the line?'
Answer: 'Yes.'
Question: 'Now, is his tail following the line?'
Answer: 'No.'
Question: 'How do you know it's not?'
Answer: 'I looked behind me.'

Once the rider has observed the problem the next step is for him/her to be able to feel it without looking. In this form of questioning breakdown, the closed question with a yes or no answer is used. This is permissible as it is followed by a series of back-up questions with a specified aim. The reasoning ability or background knowledge of the pupil are not being questioned. There are many trainers, teachers and coaches who like to make this complicated, but in reality riding horses and the training of horse and rider are relatively simple arts that require dedication, discipline and feel. Success as a trainer depends on the ability to break things down into simple understandable chunks to help both horse and rider.

The riding instructor will also have to use questioning as a method of problem solving. For example, a horse appears to 'switch off' and lack energy at competitions. Rider and instructor need to try and identify why this happens, so the instructor questions the rider to try to get to the root of the problem and hence find a solution. The conversation may go like this:

Question: 'Has he always been like this?'
Answer: 'No, just at the last two competitions.'

Question: 'What is different now?'

The instructor can then run through the factors that may cause the horse's behaviour to change, for example:

- the weather;
- the stable management;
- is the test at the competition of the same complexity?
- has the horse displayed any signs of ill health?

If perhaps the only differentiating factor is that the test is more complex, this allows the reasoning process to progress:

- Why are the more difficult tests taxing the horse more?
- Is it a rider problem?

Ultimately the problem is probably both physical and mental and it is the trainer's task to endeavour to help the rider through both of these difficult areas.

Constructive feedback

Pupils require feedback as part of the teaching and learning process; it encourages self-awareness and development. Critical comment, given correctly, will help pupils improve their performance (Fig. 4.2).

Start with the positive – it helps pupils to tell them what they have done well; it also ensures that you have their attention. For example, 'I like the way you checked the tack for safety'.

Be specific – try to pinpoint what the person actually did rather than just give a general comment such as 'excellent' or 'poor'. For example, 'Your handling of the horse while you fitted the tack was safe'; 'You fitted the throatlash too tightly – it should allow the width of a hand between the cheekbone'.

Suggest ways of changing behaviour to get a better result. Pupils cannot change unless you give them guidance, so do not say 'You are no good because you caught the horse in the teeth'; give advice to help them improve their performance, for example, 'Try to allow more with the hands over the fence so that you do not get left behind the movement'.

Own the feedback

Feedback that starts with 'You are . . .' gives the impression that this is

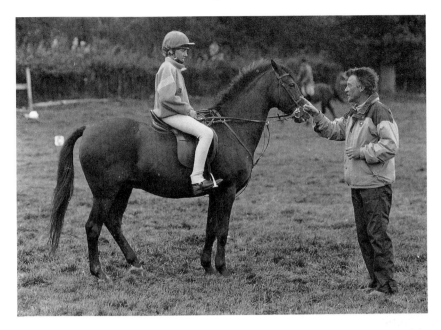

Fig. 4.2 Feedback is part of the teaching and learning process. Start with the positive and take care that your body language is not more aggressive than you mean to be.

an opinion held by everybody. Saying 'In my opinion...' ensures that the teacher takes responsibility for what he/she is saying.

Leave the pupil with a choice

Insisting on change may be met with resistance while suggestions of ways of improving performance are more likely to be accepted. For example, 'If you want to turn out to a really high standard, you could polish the buckles on the headcollar'.

Assessment

Assessment is an important component of the learning process. It can be used by the teacher to monitor progress as well as achievement and also serves to ensure that pupils are aware of their own progress. Indeed, assessment should be of more use to the pupil than to the teacher. Some of the reasons for assessment include:

- to assess progress/achievement;
- to give feedback on progress;
- to diagnose weaknesses;
- to discover strengths;

- to assess the effectiveness of the teaching;
- motivation;
- to give information for qualification and certification;
- to select for groups or courses;
- to provide feedback for parents.

Forms of assessment

Every time we meet and talk to other people we make some form of assessment about them. This informal assessment is known as formative assessment and is used every time you teach pupils in order to provide them with ongoing feedback. The most useful form of assessment for the riding teacher is criterion-referenced assessment which measures the ability of the pupil to perform tasks to predetermined standards of performance. In other words the teacher assesses if a person is competent to nationally devised standards such as British Horse Society Qualifications or National Vocational Qualifications. Criterion-referenced assessment is useful for:

- helping the trainee to learn;
- diagnosing strengths and weaknesses;
- determining if the trainee has the required knowledge and skills;
- establishing what the trainee has learnt;
- giving credit for competency;
- helping the trainee take responsibility for his/her own learning through self-assessment;
- giving a clear indication of what is required in assessments.

Traditionally the riding instructor has been involved in practical teaching, but there is an increasing requirement for written assessments, which may cover practical aspects of riding, teaching and stable management as well as more theoretical aspects such as horse health, anatomy and physiology.

Assignments

Assignments are tasks and exercises structured by the teacher and undertaken by the pupil with access to reference material. The outcome of the assignment, in other words what the pupil has to accomplish, is clearly stated. An assignment must be legible, complete, technically accurate and feasible. It may also have to be presented by a certain deadline. Assignments are frequently used to back up theoretical areas of teaching that cannot be covered in practice, such as foaling when there are no brood mares available.

Projects

Projects tend to be more practical in nature and involve the gathering of material over a period of time and an analysis of that material. Projects tend to pull together the strands of many aspects of the teaching material and are sometimes referred to as integrative as they integrate different subject areas. For example, the project may be to prepare a horse for a specific competitive goal. This would involve an assessment of the horse to establish the goal, developing and implementing a feeding and fitness programme, training the horse for the specific discipline and monitoring its health during the programme.

Tips for encouraging learning skills

Deal with getting it wrong – part of the learning process is making mistakes and getting it wrong. It is better to be doing something and doing it wrong (a positive mistake) than doing nothing at all.

Think a lot – thinking, understanding and remembering are just as important for practical task. You cannot just rely on 'feel'.

Practise – acquiring skills demands practice; a horse cannot get better at doing medium trot unless he does medium trot. The quality may be poor at first but will improve with practice.

Question – keep asking 'why', 'what if' and 'how'. Thinking and understanding is central to effective learning.

Effective listening

Regardless of the learning style of a pupil, effective listening is a very important communication skill. The following mnemonic may help:

L   look forward – read up before the lesson and identify possible questions.
I   ideas – try to note down any important ones.
S   signals – identify key ideas, such as 'This is important...' or 'Remember this...'.
T   take part – be active and attentive.
E   explore – ask questions.
N   notes – take notes as an *aide mémoire*.

Rider fitness

The fitness of a horse is of paramount importance. Unfortunately riders have tended not to place such emphasis on their own fitness. Their level of fitness will determine what they are physically capable of doing during a lesson. It is easy for the teacher who is accustomed to riding every day to overestimate the fitness of novice and infrequent riders. Once riders become tired they will stop learning; indeed they are more likely to make mistakes and lose confidence. On the other hand, riders who are fit may feel that they have underachieved unless they work quite hard during a lesson.

Fit riders will be:

- able to ride for longer;
- less tired;
- able to enjoy themselves more;
- healthier.

The level of fitness a rider requires will depend on what he/she wants to do; race riding or three day eventing requires a rider to be very fit while pleasure riding does not. The teacher needs to be aware of the different needs of pupils and tailor the demands of the lessons to suit the individual.

There are five components of physical fitness which are well recognized when training horses. They are also important to develop when training riders:

- Flexibility is the range of movement of a joint or joints. The pupils' age will affect their flexibility.
- Endurance is the capacity to perform prolonged low intensity activity without getting tired. This may not be as important to the show jumper as it is to the long-distance rider.
- Speed is the time taken to co-ordinate movement of the body or parts of the body. All riders need to be able to react quickly.
- Strength is the maximum force that a muscle or muscles can generate. A certain amount of physical strength is necessary, but technique can reduce the amount required.
- Power is the maximum force that can be generated by the muscles in the shortest possible time. Speed and power often go together.

It is possible for a person to be well developed in one area and quite weak in another and while the importance of each component varies according to the demands of the discipline, all riders require some development of each physical fitness component.

Each rider will respond differently to the fitness training that will be built into a series of riding lessons. This is due to:

- heredity – different physical and mental properties will have been inherited from the parents;
- maturity – children and young people are still growing and developing and there will be less spare energy for training;
- nutrition – an adequate well balanced diet is important for top performers;
- rest and recovery – riders involved in tough training schedules and frequent competitions will get tired and need rest and recovery. Some will cope better than others and the trainer must be aware of this;
- the present level of fitness – this will dictate how quickly the rider can progress. A complete beginner will not have any of the riding muscles developed and will have to progress slowly.

The rider's muscles, tendons and ligaments need time to adjust to the stresses caused by riding. Just as with horses, the body adapts slowly and trying to rush the process can cause discomfort, pain and even injury. Initially the teacher must work within the fitness levels of the rider. Gradually increasing the demands allows the body to adapt to the new activity or level of training so that the rider's body:

- has better circulation, respiration and heart function;
- improved strength and endurance;
- tougher bones, tendons and ligaments.

Regardless of the fitness of the rider and the content of the lesson remember that work should be followed by rest and recovery and that intensive sessions should be followed by a more relaxed one. Riders can become bored with lessons so it is important for the teacher to vary the content and style of the sessions as far as is possible, to maintain motivation and to stimulate interest.

Warm up
It is important that both horse and rider warm up effectively and while we pay conscientious attention to warming up the horse we rarely bother about the rider. An effective warm up should:

- warm up the whole body to raise muscle and blood temperature and stretch the muscles and connective tissue;
- be directly related to the activity to be performed;
- be suited to the individual participant;
- combine intensity and duration without being tiring;
- take place at the start of a session.

Generally as we take the horse through his warm up programme the rider also warms up. There is, however, one important aspect that is not taken care of by riding the horse, and it is one that the athlete considers vital – stretching. For efficient function, stretching exercises which work the muscles used when the body is in action should be incorporated into the warm up. Begin at the top and work down to cover:

- neck and shoulders
- arms and chest
- lower back and stomach
- groin and hips
- thigh
- lower leg and ankle.

Cool down
It is equally important to cool down after a session is over. Stiffness (in horse and rider) may be prevented by continuing to move the affected muscles in a gentle rhythmic state. Stretching exercises can also ease muscles that have worked hard and become tight. Warm showers, baths or massage may also aid recovery unless the rider has suffered a strain or a sprain.

Flexibility
Due to the nature of their sport riders often become strong and lose some flexibility. Stretching is the key to developing flexibility. Static stretching involves a slow sustained movement in which the muscle is lengthened and then held in position for 15–30 seconds. Each stretch should be followed by relaxation and the procedure repeated several times. Stretching can be used as part of a warm up or cool down; stretching after a session helps relaxation and recovery. The muscles should be warmed up before stretching starts and the stretching should never be painful. Straining may damage the muscles. However there should be enough stretch for pull to be felt in the bulky central

part of the muscle. As the feeling of stretching decreases, the stretch can go a little further. The rider must breathe calmly and regularly and not be tempted to hold his/her breath. The exercises should be chosen for the individual rider and take place before the rider gets on the horse. The following examples can be used for most riders:

Neck (Fig. 4.3) – slowly move the chin down towards the top of the chest, hold this position then push the chin up and forwards, then hold. Keep the back straight. Do not circle the head around the neck.

Shoulders and chest – gently bring arms together behind the head as shown in Fig. 4.4. Bend sideways at the waist and try to pull the elbow down to the floor. Keep the arms behind the head.

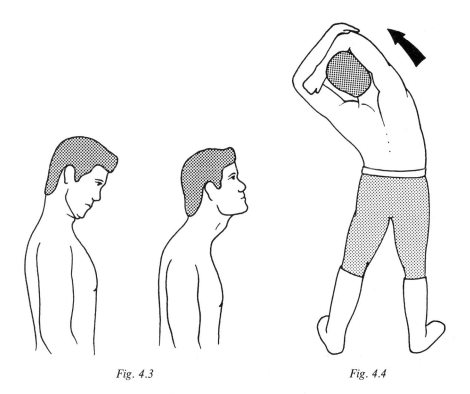

Fig. 4.3   Fig. 4.4

Arms, shoulders and chest (Fig. 4.5) – hold the arms extended up above the head with the palms together. Stretch the arms upwards and slightly backwards at the same time as breathing in.

Arms and shoulders (Fig. 4.6) – with the arms behind the head, hold the elbow of one arm with the hand of the other arm and gently pull the elbow across behind the head.

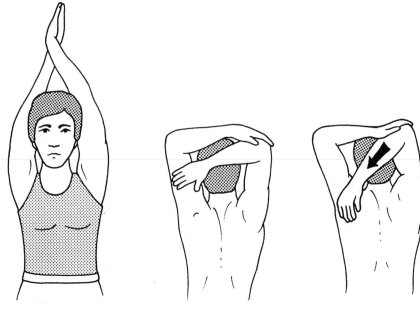

Fig. 4.5   *Fig. 4.6*

5 Lesson Planning

There are many different ways to teach – you may be an extrovert enthusiast or a quiet, firm organizer. Remember that however knowledgeable and enthusiastic you are, the effectiveness of your teaching will depend on good planning and sound practice.

Initially teaching can be quite an unnerving situation and the trainee or newly qualified teacher can run into problems. Many of these problems are not to do with personality, control or knowledge, but boil down to lack of preparation. If the lessons are part of a series, each lesson should be organized on the basis of the previous lesson. During each lesson try to assess what is going well, what is going badly and what is needed for next time.

A good teacher is not afraid of making mistakes; indeed, it has been said that a good instructor is not someone who does it right all the time, but someone who can recognize when things are going wrong and puts it right next time. This means that a series of lessons which have been designed to cover a certain syllabus may have to be modified after a couple of lessons. The novice instructor may benefit from keeping a notebook as a reminder of which activities went well and which went badly and how these could be monitored.

Spend time preparing the lesson. Concentrate on:

- safety – identify possible danger areas;
- motivation – why is the group here, what are their short and long term goals?
- learning – what do they want to learn?
- organization – ensure the lesson runs smoothly, for example, set up and check equipment before the lesson.

At all times be considerate to the needs of your pupils. Spend some time getting to know them (Fig. 5.1), be polite and respectful of their opinions so that you share the learning with them. This is important

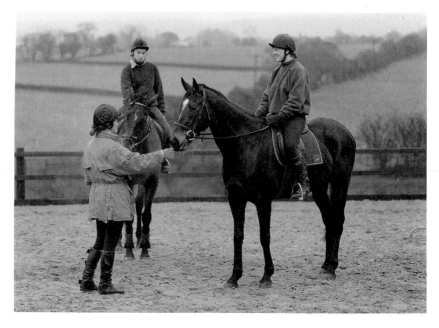

Fig. 5.1 Spend some time getting to know your pupils.

for mature novice riders as the sense of partnership encourages them to remain involved and promotes a feeling of fulfilment as well as enjoyment.

Riders who are purposefully employed throughout the lesson will learn almost without trying. Follow these guidelines:

- Identify the modification of their riding technique that is needed. This should be a modification that will help them, not one that you think that they ought to have.
- Check that your pupils understand why this modification is needed and in what way it will be helpful.
- Develop the correct technique in a situation where the rider is not under pressure.
- As soon as possible put the technique into practice and monitor improvement.

In groups of mixed ability and experience it can be difficult to follow these guidelines; thought must be given to sub-dividing the group or finding an exercise that will be beneficial to all.

Timing

Always start and finish on time and allow sufficient time to warm up and cool down both horse and rider. Remember you are teaching and helping riders, not just presenting a series of exercises. Be flexible: while it is useful to try to plan how long to spend on each exercise, you may find that the riders pick it up very quickly or perhaps rather slowly. Give equal time to all pupils in the lesson so that pupils do not feel any unfairness or discrimination. Be aware of any differences in age, gender, ability or ethnicity which may influence the needs of your pupils. Good teachers are able to adapt their practice to accommodate everybody.

Planning a lesson

Preparation

Before helping pupils to learn new skills, it is important to prepare their lesson. In order to do this you need to establish what the pupils know and can do already and what they want to learn. When you are planning a lesson first focus on what you want your pupils to be able to do and how well they should be able to do it and then set the objectives of the lesson. Riders must understand what is expected of them and how quickly this might be achieved. A clear statement of the results you require will enable you to:

- plan the instruction – work out how best to achieve the objectives;
- help your pupils understand what is expected of them;
- assess progress – have you achieved your aim?

If you find it difficult to state your objectives clearly try breaking it down:

- Action – what will your pupils be able to do at the end of the lesson or series of lessons?
- Standards – how well will they be able to do it?
- Conditions – under what conditions/on what sort of horse will they be able to do it?

Example
Action – the rider will be able to jump.

Standard – a course of fences no more than 3 ft 3 in (1 m) high.
Conditions – on a schooled, quiet horse.

This makes the teacher focus on 'What do I want the pupil to do?'
rather than 'What am I going to teach the pupil?'. At all times your
objectives must be realistic and achievable. This can be ascertained in
discussion with the pupils; you need to establish their previous
experience, what their goals are, how long you have and how many
pupils will be in the lesson.

Content

Having ascertained the needs of the pupils, the content of the lesson
depends on what to teach, in what order and with what facilities.
Thinking in detail about the content of the lesson will help you plan
what the pupils will do at each stage of the lesson. Information should
be delivered in easily digested chunks, emphasizing the essential
information or key points that are vital to learning the skill.

Next decide the correct order in which to teach the chunks to make
learning easier. For skills other than very simple ones it is very
important to break the result down into a series of learning steps and
to get your pupil to perform part of the skill or answer questions at
each step. Usually there will be natural breaks in the skill that will
allow you to get the pupil to do one bit at a time.

For example, the learning steps in a jumping lesson might be:

(1) Introduction.
(2) Warm up on the flat.
(3) Jump a cross pole from trot.
(4) Jump a small upright from canter.
(5) Jump a small ascending oxer.
(6) Plan a course.
(7) Jump a course.
(8) Summary, feedback and homework.

Having decided on the learning steps the next stage in preparing the
lesson is to decide what key points to emphasize when teaching each
learning step. The way to do this is to identify anything in each
learning step that may cause your pupil difficulty. To make learning
more effective only identify key points that are vital to learning or to
safety. Too many points will lose their impact.

Example
Learning step – jump a small upright from canter.
Key points – quality of canter
            – approach
            – position over fence
            – get away.

Usually the best sequence in which to teach the learning steps is the logical way that you have approached the skill. However, you may decide to deal with a difficult point first to get it out of the way. This means that you can then teach the whole skill, step by step, without having to interrupt the flow to deal with the difficult part.

How to teach the content
When you introduce yourself you will also outline the lesson content in such a way that it is relevant to the pupils. Set the context by asking the pupils why they would like these skills and then suggesting how these skills will help them. The content of the lesson should be taught in manageable chunks remembering that learning by doing is the basic principle that should be applied throughout any lesson.

'I do it normal   – demonstrate complete skill;
I do it slow   – show it bit by bit;
You do it with me   – pupil learns one bit at a time;
Then off you go'   – pupil puts it together.

Choose the right technique for the specific content of the lesson, taking into account the facilities you have available. Choosing the most appropriate technique will:

● help the pupil master the skill;
● ensure that the objectives of the lesson are achieved;
● make the role of the teacher both easier, more successful and more rewarding.

Choosing your method
Teaching a person to ride cannot be taught by lectures or simulation, but some aspects of stable management, for example, can be learned peacefully at the pupil's own rate from a book at home. Table 5.1 is a guide suggesting which methods match the teaching objective.

Table 5.1   A guide to matching the teaching objective.

When your objective is to teach a skill choose from:

- Demonstration
- Discovery method
- Individual practice
- Lesson-demonstration

When your objective is to impart knowledge choose from:

- Case study/projects
- Discussion
- Lectures
- Private study
- Tutorial

When your objective is to change attitudes choose from:

- Role play
- Simulation
- Discussion
- Tutorials

The method you choose will be influenced by your own preferences and those of your pupils as well as the facilities available (Table 5.2). Using a variety of methods generates a sense of curiosity, fun and excitement in both pupil and teacher and prevents learning becoming dull and stale. Remember, verbally-given information is the hardest to learn, people learn at different rates and learn best when they have some control over the pace of the learning. Everybody is anxious about failure and needs reassurance, you do not learn unless you are told you have made the correct response. The best way to learn is through activity, by actually using the knowledge or practising the skill.

The most commonly used teaching techniques include:

- demonstration followed by practice;
- demonstration followed by questions;
- demonstration with the pupil copying the teacher;
- verbal demonstrations with questions and/or talkback;
- written instructions;
- question and answer.

Throughout the lesson a different method may be used for each of the identified learning steps, if this is necessary. A look at the key points at each step will help you decide which method would be most appropriate. If the key point is easy to observe, a demonstration technique may be applicable, but if the point is more difficult to see clearly and perhaps involves an element of risk, then verbal demonstration may be used.

Table 5.2 Putting over the content. Task: lungeing a horse.

Method	What happens	Examples
Observing	Demonstrations	Lungeing a horse Safe procedures Rapport with the horse
Listening	Lecture with overhead projector	Correct equipment for horse and trainer. Logical steps under various circumstances
Translating words and diagrams	Write an assignment	Lungeing the young horse – the schoolmaster for teaching – the horse for improvement
Questioning	After demonstration	Problems encountered Varying methods Prevailing circumstances
Recording	Take notes	Safety – correct procedure Further training
Experiencing/practising	Opportunities by practice	Preparing the horse for lungeing Correct procedure for holding the rein How to start and stop
Memorizing	Student to give lecture or demonstration	Assessment
Understanding	Ask about purpose Problems Assess work	Compare different horses Why lunge? Problems encountered Temperament, time, fitness
Assessing performance standards	Self assessment Assess others	Compare horse at different stages – has he improved? With the trainer or the student
Identifying and correcting errors	How to correct others' and/or horses' faults	Identifying faults and good points to establish the horse's own capacity

Throughout the lesson adopt a helpful style, breaking the instruction down into easily learned steps, using techniques that make the pupil think. Correct errors at an appropriate time and encourage the pupil to ask questions. Remember that during the lesson you may have to remind pupils of the incentives to learn, which may include:

- achievement;
- master a skill;
- more fun;
- reward.

Pupils should always be encouraged – a positive comment is better than a negative one, e.g. 'Carry your hands a little higher' not 'Don't carry your hands so low'. Be quick to congratulate pupils and to remind them what has been achieved. It is also essential to follow up the lesson with regular checks to ensure that your pupil continues to perform effectively.

Writing a lesson plan

All lessons should follow a pattern including an introduction followed by the learning part where information or techniques are introduced and then practised, and finally there should be a summary.

Preparing a lesson plan will help you achieve the objectives in the time available. A plan will also help you overcome nervousness, improve your confidence and act as a guide to what you and the pupils will be doing at a specific time during the lesson. Make sure that you have the right equipment and resources – a lesson plan could differ greatly if you were in a field compared with an indoor school.

- Objective – always write the objective at the top of the plan; this will help keep you on track.
- Introduction – you may be nervous at this stage and writing your introduction out in detail will help overcome this.
- Learning steps – write each learning step in bold writing that stands out on the page. Make very brief notes on the key points. It may be helpful to note the times for each step, this will help ensure that you cover everything. Note the teaching method to be used and any teaching aids needed.
- Summary – plan the summary to end on a positive note. Check the key points and link them to the next lesson to allow the pupil to progress.

Example lesson plan
Objective – pupils will be able to tack up a horse for lungeing.

Step	Key points	Technique and aids
Introduction (4 minutes)	Relax pupils	
	Names	First names if not known
	Objective	At the end of the lesson pupils will be able to tack up a horse for lungeing
	Scope and purpose	Explain why we lunge horses and the type of horse they will be expected to deal with.
	Previous experience	Who has done this before?
	Motivate	Ask them the uses of lungeing
Collect equipment (4 minutes)	Identify	Name and describe the lungeing equipment
Catch and tie up horse (2 minutes)	In stable	Teacher catches horse Explains safety protocol
Handle equipment (10 minutes)	Fitting	Teacher fits lungeing gear
	Safety	Checking of equipment Handling of horse
	Remove equipment	Teacher takes off tack
Practice (10 minutes)	Recognize correct fit	Pupils fit lungeing gear, talk teacher through procedure
Summary (4 minutes)	Recap purpose	Ask if any questions
	Key points	Ask specific questions, e.g.
	Handle horse	When?
	Fitting	How?
	Removing equipment	How?
	Safety	Why?
	Homework	Practise tomorrow
	Next session	Lungeing

Choosing training aids

Training aids should be used if they will help the pupil learn. Written aids are useful as:

- memory joggers
- reference material
- instructions
- a means to reduce explanation.

Three dimensional aids such as models or mock ups can:

- allow practice with out-of-season skills, for example lungeing can be practised without a horse by tying the lunge rein to a door or by the pupils lungeing each other;
- reveal hidden detail.

Presentation aids such as boards, flip charts, overhead projectors, television and video can:

- clarify and reduce explanation;
- summarize or reinforce information;
- record the pupils' input.

Practical teaching

The first time you teach a horse and rider you are unlikely to have a well defined lesson plan as you will not be familiar with the combination. This first session is therefore going to consist of an initial evaluation, followed by some work on identified problem areas. It is helpful to use the following guidelines:

(1) Introduce yourself, find out the pupils' names and use them. The idea is to try to relax the pupils by getting them to do something as quickly as possible. Explain to the pupils what the aim of the lesson is and how you hope to achieve that, in other words how the lesson will progress. Emphasize any safety points such as the rules of the school. Find out as much as possible about the horse and rider, this will help you assess their existing skills. Gain the pupils' interest and attention so that you can motivate them to want to learn.

(2) Stand back and evaluate the horses' paces, balance, acceptance of the bridle and standard of training.

(3) Study the riders' positions, use of the aids and methods of schooling.

(4) You may ride the horse, normally to check that what you have seen is reflected in what you feel.

(5) Explain to the riders what you have seen and felt and what you feel it would be best to improve. If you want to demonstrate a point make sure the pupils are positioned so that they can see clearly what you are doing. Try to exaggerate or slow down complex aids so that the pupils can see exactly what is happening.

(6) Give yourself one or two aims in 30 minutes; you will probably want to do more. Ask questions to get the pupils thinking and ensure that they have grasped one stage before moving onto the next. Let your pupils know how they are doing, and if an error occurs, stop the pupils, ask them what mistake has happened and then between you work out why the error occurred. Then you can ask the pupil to put it right and carry on. Few people can concentrate on riding the horse, listen to you, analyse a mistake and then put it right all at once. If the pupils remain confused you may have to demonstrate the point to clarify it. It is nearly always better for pupils to work out what has gone wrong and put it right themselves than for you to step in and put it right for them.

Put across the key points with real emphasis and check that the pupils have understood by questioning them. However, do not let the lesson turn into a lecture; keep demonstrations and explanations short. Each pupil will learn at a different rate so adapt the pace of your lesson to suit the pupil.

(7) Be flexible if something does not work; be prepared to find another way to achieve your objective.

(8) Ask the riders which part of the lesson they felt was of most benefit to the horse.

(9) If you are to teach the riders again, make a plan for the next lesson and suggest homework.

Remember, perfection is not achieved in one lesson, to make progress is sufficient. In addition the pupils must finish the lesson feeling that they have achieved something. If you are observing a lesson or teaching someone to teach take note of the following points:

- Could you hear?
- Did the teacher introduce him-/herself?
- Were the explanations clear and the demonstrations accurate?
- Was the lesson planned, well prepared and structured?
- Was some praise given?
- Were useful corrections given?
- Was progress towards improvement started?

Features of successful instruction (Table 5.3)

Your aim as a teacher is to achieve results, in other words to get your pupil to perform a certain skill to the required level. Success is easier to achieve if the teacher follows the following guidelines:

Table 5.3 Checklist for successful instruction.

	Prepare
	Focus on results – set objective
	Plan learning steps
	Identify key points
	Check facilities and equipment
	Instruct
Instructor style	Show interest and confidence
	Treat pupil as a mature person
	Encourage questions and discussion
Introducing	Establish required result
	Gain pupil's interest and attention
	Find out past experience
Showing how	Give clear demonstration at each step
	Emphasize key points
	Hold learner's attention
Helping to learn	Give adequate time for practice
	Inform pupil of progress
	Spot errors and help pupil to correct
	Check
At end of lesson	Can pupil do the task to the required standard?
Following up	Is pupil continuing up to standard?

- Preparing and organizing – think out the lesson first so that you have a clear picture of the result you want and the learning steps involved in achieving this. Then write it down.
- Introducing – get the lesson off to a good start so that the pupil is clear about the purpose of the lesson and how you will achieve it.
- Showing how – give clear, well presented demonstration and explanation at each step.
- Helping to learn – the pupil must be involved and given adequate opportunity to practise each step so that he/she can overcome any difficulties experienced as they arise.
- Instructor style – the teacher is critical to success; if you are interested and confident the pupil will become confident as well. Always give constructive criticism.
- Following up – always check that the pupil continues to perform the skill correctly; do not let the standards slip.

Developing your style

The style you adopt during a lesson will affect how much your pupils learn and how effective the lesson is. You should try to minimize the amount of material that you feed to the pupils and maximize the amount that they are made to think.

- Be confident – if you are thoroughly familiar with the task you will appear confident.
- Be prepared – have a lesson plan and all the necessary equipment ready.
- Show your pupils that you think it is important for them to be successful and that you are confident in their ability to be successful.
- Involve the pupils through practice and questioning without making them feel under pressure.
- Encourage them to assess the quality of their work; this develops a self-critical approach to their learning.
- Ask them to explain why they think their work is of a particular quality. This gives you the opportunity to correct any misconceptions they may have.
- Encourage pupils to ask you for help when they have a problem; this allows them to take some control of their learning.
- Treat pupils as mature individuals and never patronize them.
- Praise good work and effort.
- Be patient with those experiencing difficulties.
- Encourage questions and discussion, giving prompt and helpful answers.

6 The Plan in Action

Having set the goals and drawn up your lesson plan you now have to implement that plan, in other words you have to teach the lesson and try to achieve the goals. How often have you overheard lessons like the following?

Mr Sergeant

'No, no, no . . . , that looks awful . . . What ever do you think you are doing? . . . Unless you do better than that you'll never pass any exams . . . More bend . . . For goodness sake, can't you remember anything I tell you? . . . No, that's not good enough, do it again . . . No, I've told you a thousand times, don't cross your hand over. Don't you ever listen? . . . Repeat that and get it right this time . . . That was terrible . . . For crying out loud, don't you want to do it properly? . . . then pay attention and do as you are told . . . Don't be so stupid . . . Do try and think before you act. God gave you a brain, why don't you use it? . . . Oh, you are useless . . . .'

Mrs Goodbody

'Oh, well done Sam . . . That was lovely June . . . Well not quite right but never mind . . . Splendid Maria . . . Jolly good Hilary . . . Oh, bad luck dear. Let's try it again shall we? . . . Oh, love, that was really good . . . Oh, hurrah Dawn . . . Keep it up everybody . . . Isn't this fun? . . . Pat your horse June, let him know he's done well. You can give yourself a pat too because you deserve it . . . Oh, well tried. That was a good attempt . . . .'

Mrs Busy

'Right everybody, sorry I'm late. Check your tack, mount and warm up your horses. I'm just going to grab a coffee . . . OK folks? Jolly good. Just go over that exercise I gave you last week. I'll only be a moment, got to make a phone call . . . OK everybody? Sorry that took a bit longer than I expected. Never mind. Right, I'll show you a new exercise. Let me hop on your horse Nicola. Look, this is how it goes. Now you all try it. Oh, dear there's someone ringing the office bell, back in a tick....'

Captain Drill

'Ride from the front – tell off by fours ... numbers one to four are number one ride, numbers five to eight are number two ride. Number one ride, prove. As you were ... I shall say "Ride – Walk – March" and on the word "March", not before, I want each of you to make your horse walk on promptly and smoothly. Ride – Walk – March ... Eve, shorten your reins ... Prepare to trot. Ride, ter-rot ... inclining across the school in rides. Number one ride, right incline....'

Cathy Peat

'Right, get on then, check your tack and on the right rein go large ... Trot on then ... OK, ride walk ... leading files trotting to the rear of the ride, commence ... Next ... Next ... Next ... follow on ... Right, whole ride trot on. Leading files cantering to the rear of the ride, commence ... Next ... Wrong leg ... Next ... If you can't do it just join the rear. Next ... Whole ride trot and walk ... Keep your spacing ... Right, quit and cross your stirrups ... Leading files trotting to the rear of the – oh, let's change the rein first. Nearly forgot. Right, change the rein ... Now, leading files trotting to the rear of the ride. Commence....'

Rod Cathgoe

'Good Lyn, that's nice but a little more impulsion. No, not speed, impulsion. That's better ... Well done Megan, you are getting a nice tune out of that horse ... Philip, be careful you are not getting back into that old habit of bringing the hand across the neck. Think open rein. Now in the next corner "Open the door", that's much better ... Whole ride, in your own time, end the exercise you are doing, walk and form a ride on the right rein with Lyn as leading file. Well done everyone, that was better than a week ago. Still some important points to work on, but it is going well ... Now both you and your horses are warmed up I would like to introduce you to a new exercise. The exercise is called Caragula. It is one that I find useful when suppling up some horses and it's not too difficult to master. Ride, prepare to turn in and halt. Ride, turn in and halt....'

I am sure that you recognize some of the faults that you and other riding instructors may have. Bearing these in mind, let us look at the implementation of some lesson plans. You have to consider:

- the riders – ability and number in the lesson;
- the horses – age and standard of training;
- the facilities;
- the time available;
- equipment;
- time of day.

Horses and riders are all individuals and must be treated as such. Bearing this in mind, the teacher must be able to react and teach the pupils and horses in front of him/her, even if it means deviating from the lesson plan. The following examples give you some idea of how the lesson plan works in action and include:

- the novice lesson
- lunge lesson
    - for the novice
    - for the advanced
- flat work
    - individual Pony Club child
    - adult working at medium dressage level
    - class lesson
- riding club lesson
- jumping lesson
    - the young horse; lessons 1 and 2
    - the class jumping lesson; novice and advanced grid work
    - advanced individual show jumping lesson
    - cross country schooling; novice and advanced.

The novice lesson

The aim of the novice lesson is to build the rider's confidence and develop his/her position and feel (Fig. 6.1). In this case the pupil is a seven-year-old girl who has been having weekly lessons at a riding school. After four to six lessons on the leading rein she is ready to have a go at riding on her own; this lesson is still on a one-to-one basis and is her first lesson off the leading rein. Ideally the teacher

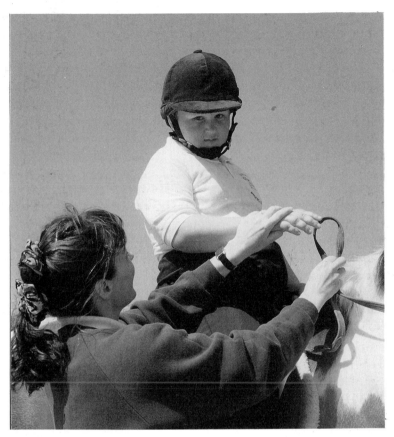

Fig. 6.1 The aim of the novice lesson is to build confidence. (*Courtesy:* Riding for the Disabled Association)

should be the same each time, provided that the child is confident with that teacher.

Start on the lead rein to check that the child is confident and in control. She should be able to start and stop, make turns and ride one long side of the school in trot, but she may not yet have mastered rising trot. Check by discussion and questioning that the pupil has understood everything to date. Make any appropriate positional corrections and in particular check that her application of the aids is correct.

When the lead rein is first released, it is important that the teacher keeps reasonably close to the pony; this gives the child confidence and means that you can hear what she is saying. You are also able to step in should a potentially hazardous situation arise. *Never* leave alone a child who is nervous; if she says she can't, do not make her. Encourage her by introducing the task that she is frightened of in the smallest possible chunks.

Again check that the child is in control, perhaps by giving her markers to work to. If she cannot ride the pony to the marker, discuss why and try to help her achieve this goal in today's session. On the first occasion that the child is riding alone *do not* become too ambitious, for example the lesson is *not* a failure if the child does not trot on her own. Turns, transitions, circles, changes of direction are all achievements and should be praised as such. However, if the child is really keen to trot she should be allowed to try, but keep the trot short and stay close to the pony.

Try from the outset to involve your rider in how the pony feels. Give her some responsibility and *never* allow a child to be rough or abusive to a pony. Establish a caring attitude from the start.

It is possible to do all this in a ride situation providing that there are enough helpers. The helpers must be involved in the lesson and feel part of this learning situation. The instructor should keep a written record of the rider's progress, what she has done and which pony she has ridden. This enables future plans to be developed and, should the child change the teacher or move to another riding school, she has a record that she can take with her.

Lunge lesson

For the novice

The aim of giving a novice rider a lunge lesson is to build confidence, to establish a safe, correct seat and to enable the pupil to progress (Fig. 6.2). The degree of progression will depend on the individual.

The pupil and instructor should agree a series of lessons from which the pupil can progress, for example, to join a ride of other novice riders. The type of pupil will vary. For this scenario let us consider a middle-aged housewife whose children ride and who feels like taking on a challenge. This means that the client has a basic knowledge of horses and knows what it takes to make an average rider. Today's lesson plan is for lesson four and the goal is to develop the rising trot. Some work in trot has been carried out in the previous three lessons. The lunge lesson should last no more than 30 minutes.

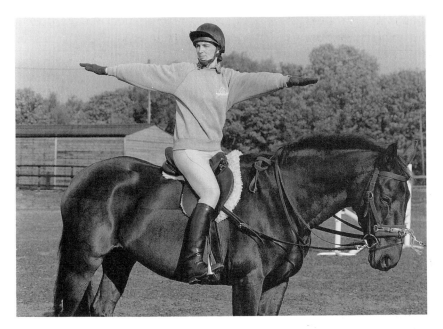

Fig. 6.2 Exercises can be used to promote confidence and to develop the correct position.

Lesson plan

Check the tack. The horse should be fitted with either a breastplate or a neck strap.

0–5 minutes: Work in the horse for five minutes, without the rider, on both reins. Encourage the rider to participate by telling her how the horse is going and what you are looking for. Help her to observe the horse and feedback her observations to you. Observation and 'feel' go hand in hand, especially when lungeing horses. The horse should be worked without side reins initially; the side reins can then be put on and fitted to suit that particular horse. The rider should always mount and dismount with the side reins unclipped or unbuckled.

5–10 minutes: The rider can then mount and the stirrups can be adjusted as necessary. Revise the rider's position in walk and include some transitions to halt on both reins; this should last 5–10 minutes. The control of the horse should be dual: from your voice and from the rider's aids. This work is ideal for creating maximum communication between pupil and teacher. It is essential to compare the feel that the rider has, from lesson to lesson, to ensure that progress is made each time.

10–15 minutes: Trot work can then be introduced. First of all the rider should be in sitting trot and holding either the pommel of the saddle or the breastplate. This gives the rider security and allows her to feel the rhythm of the trot. The reins should be knotted underneath the breastplate or neck strap for later use. The periods of trot should be short, perhaps three circles and then some walk. Always ask the rider if she is tired and if keen to go on for longer this can be negotiated. Remember that her riding muscles will not be fit and that if she becomes tired it will create tension and discomfort.

15–25 minutes: Progress to introduce the concept of rising trot. If one method does not succeed be prepared to try another. Do not forget to praise the rider whenever progress is made, even if it is only for two or three strides. This part of the lesson should last about ten minutes.

25–30 minutes: Leave five minutes at the end of the lesson in order to cool down the horse and the pupil and to debrief the pupil and give some homework. This could include some floor exercises, reading or watching a video – anything to encourage study and involvement from your pupil.

Remember to change the rein every 8–10 minutes and to let the rider help with the manoeuvre. Lunge lessons can be strenuous for novice riders and some feel nervous when asked to relinquish the reins. Develop sufficient rapport so that your pupil trusts you by being sensitive to these potential problems.

The advanced lunge lesson

The aim of the advanced lunge lesson is to promote the depth of seat, suppleness and feel of experienced riders. Again, a 30 minute session is ample. Your pupil may be working for the BHSI (British Horse Society Instructor) examination, perhaps he/she is a good practical rider but lacks depth of seat and finesse. Regular lungeing has been recommended to enhance the normal riding and teaching regime. In this case the rider is fit and, in order for the lesson to be of benefit, the horse must be well trained and a good mover that uses his back well in order to give the rider a chance to develop a deep seat.

The horse should be worked in as before, initially without the side reins and then with the side reins. If work in canter is to be included in the lesson, canter the horse before mounting the rider to check the horse's obedience and cooperation. This is particularly important if the teacher is not familiar with the horse. The warm up should last 5–8 minutes, during which the pupil is encouraged to observe the horse and to initiate discussion of his responsiveness and way of going. The rider is then mounted and the side reins attached. In this case, as the rider and trainer are familiar with each other, the lesson is started without the stirrups but the reins are kept. The trainer must be careful to study the rider's position and posture and make adjustments or suggest exercises that are specifically chosen for that particular rider. Transition work will be part of the lesson, both from pace to pace and within the pace, to enable the rider to develop his/her balance further. The reins may be given away whenever the trainer is satisfied that the horse is sufficiently settled. As before the rein should be changed every 8–10 minutes.

Canter is introduced with the emphasis on the rider's ability to influence the horse with the sensitivity of his/her seat. Work on collecting the canter, and transitions to and from walk are particularly beneficial. The rider should be encouraged to evaluate progress, especially with regard to the horse's movement and balance. If time permits, increasing and decreasing the circle can also help the rider become aware of any problems than can arise from lateral work. It also allows the trainer to pay close attention to the rider's straightness; this work would first be consolidated in trot.

It is often beneficial for the rider to finish the lesson with both reins and stirrups to evaluate progress. Allow time for both horse and rider to cool off, set the rider some homework and highlight special points for the rider to work on regarding his/her position.

Riding club

The scenario is an evening lesson for a group of four riding club members of mixed abilities with some positional faults, riding horses from 4 to 24 years of age. The lesson is to last 60 minutes and is to include, as its main theme, work over trotting poles. All the horses have worked over poles before, but not in this school. The equipment is limited to four 10 ft (3 m) long poles and two pairs of wings. The aim is to improve both the riders' and the horses' balance by working over four poles which are raised at one end.

Typically when asking riding club riders what they would like to do they say 'anything to make my horse better'. At first this seems very open, but by talking to them about their experiences and aspirations a goal can usually be agreed. The lesson for the above group may go something like this: the ride is asked to warm up in rising trot on the right rein in open order (Fig. 6.3). This gives the instructor a chance to see the horses work and then to comment to the rider on rhythm, tempo and rider position. After two or three circuits the riders are asked to change the rein. As the riders continue to warm up, note how

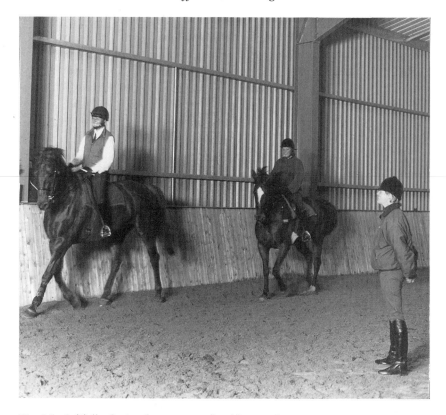

Fig. 6.3 Initially the teacher assesses the riders as they warm up.

they use the school and watch the horses' reactions to each other and to any external influences.

We then need to evaluate the canter. It is useful to put the riders on two separate circles at each end of the school; you can then stand at the edge of the school and see both groups. The riders can also canter as much or as little as their horses can manage. Advise the riders to keep looking out for the others so that they can avoid any potential dangers. The more balanced combinations should make way for the greener horses.

The walk, trot and canter will have warmed up the horses and riders and allowed the instructor to make an initial assessment. The instructor can then decide what further suppling work would be appropriate prior to the polework. We know that part of the requirement for beneficial polework will be a balanced turn and the ability to keep on a straight line, so serpentines or loops may be suitable. During these exercises, as well as correcting horse and rider, the instructor can also receive some feedback from the riders as to how they feel their horses are going. For this standard of rider and fitness of horse, a break and walking on a long rein every 10 minutes or so is beneficial. In this example there is a four-year-old horse in the ride and the rider should be given the option to drop out of any exercises should the horse feel stressed or tired.

As we progress to the polework, introduce the exercise slowly and explain that it is a valuable exercise for the young horse and that the rest can use it to improve their balance and the quality and regularity of the walk and trot (Fig. 6.4). Normally, start with the poles 4 ft 6 in (1.4 m) apart and explain why and also when it might be necessary to adjust this distance. The poles should be placed on the inside track so that all the riders can keep on the move. The exercise should be started in rising trot with a rein contact, and the riders negotiate the poles two or three times before changing the rein. For the horse the emphasis is on:

- balance
- rhythm
- straightness.

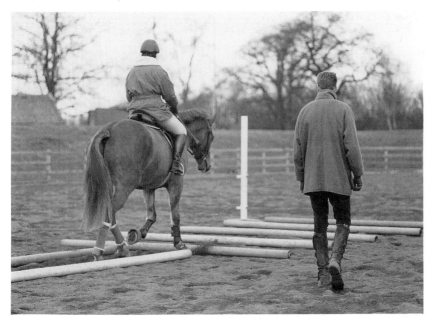

Fig. 6.4   Polework can be used to improve the balance, quality and regularity of the trot.

For the rider the emphasis is on:

- balance
- maintenance of position.

At this stage the stirrups are still at the riders' working length. Once the horses and riders are settled they can progress to the 'poised position'; they may need to shorten their stirrups a little. According to the individual standards of the riders their hands may:

- rest on the neck;
- be away from the neck with a contact;
- be away from the neck allowing stretching;
- be away from the neck allowing complete freedom.

Although the emphasis is on the poles, the rest of the work must still be monitored and the riders encouraged to maintain responsibility for their own riding pattern. The poles may then be raised slightly at alternate ends by simply resting the poles on the feet of the wings. Later you may progress to putting the ends of the poles on cups higher up the wings. If the horses become bored or begin to lack energy some work in canter may freshen them up, but usually this exercise alone is sufficiently stimulating.

Having worked on both reins through the series of exercises, encourage the riders to allow the horses to stretch down in trot and then go into walk on a long rein. The instructor can then carry out the lesson evaluation with the riders while they are on the move which will allow sufficient and proper cooling off time. Ask your riders when their horses felt at their best during the lesson and use this to suggest some homework. Encourage the riders to remain positive.

This lesson could be part of a series leading either towards developing the trot or towards jumping. If the goal is to develop the trot, subsequent lessons could include raising the poles at both ends with some work in sitting trot if the horse's back is strong enough, moving on to lengthening the distance between the poles, which is particularly beneficial for horses that find it difficult to lengthen.

If the aim is to jump, progress towards cantering over poles (Fig. 6.5), single poles at first and later a series of poles 8 ft (2.4 m) apart. Introduce placing poles for both trot and canter before and after fences, but always check that you are familiar with the distances that the poles should be set at. The instructor must be observant and

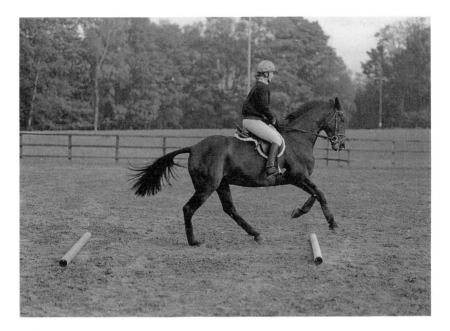

Fig. 6.5 Cantering over a series of poles; the rider has lost her balance a little.

prepared to change either the distances or the exercise if it is not having the desired effect.

Recommended distances for placing poles on the approach side of a fence would be:

- 8 ft (2.4 m) in trot;
- 9 ft (2.7 m) in canter for a bounce;
- 18 ft (5.5 m) for one stride.

On the landing side of a fence the pole should be placed 10–12 (3–3.7 m) away depending on the individual horse's stride. Instructors must be prepared to measure their own strides with a tape measure to check accuracy on a regular basis. To test yourself, close your eyes and walk the distance so that you do not anticipate and lengthen or shorten your stride to fit your guesstimate.

Remember that all exercises, but particularly jumping, are affected by the weather and the ground conditions and that you must be prepared to react to these influences.

Flat work

Individual Pony Club child

The rider is taking her Pony Club C+ test tomorrow and has come to you for a 40 minute lesson on her own horse, which is 14 years old, 15 hh and an event type. She went to two jumping competitions in the last week so the aim of the lesson is to ensure that she is confident that she can cope with the specific flat work requirements of the test.

The specific exercises that need to be covered include:

● turns and circles;
● serpentines;
● change of lead at canter through trot;
● turn on the forehand from halt;
● mounting and dismounting from both sides;
● riding with the reins in one hand;
● rising and sitting trot.

First of all ask her to warm up in walk, trot and canter on both reins. This gives the instructor the opportunity to assess horse and rider and to make some rider corrections. After the warm up ask for some lengthening of stride in trot to make sure that the horse is 'in front of the leg' before proceeding to some canter work without stirrups to deepen the rider's seat. Include some smaller circles within a 20 m circle before letting her take the stirrups back. Throughout the lesson give the horse and rider breaks in walk at 10 minute intervals – a tired rider is not a learning or effective rider. You can then move on to work on the simple change through trot; it is useful to do this from one 20 m circle to another as this makes it easier to keep the flexibility and progress to the change across the diagonal. Include both rising trot and sitting trot through the change, as you do not know which will be asked for in the test and also to ascertain which suits this horse and rider combination best.

Then include some work at sitting trot on a circle and ask for some transitions. The aim is to find the tempo that the rider is happy to cope with. We can then incorporate some work with the reins in one hand, including a change of rein, preferably from one circle to another. Progress from this to the turn on the forehand. Establish that the rider is familiar with aids and knows how to react if something goes wrong, for example the horse stepping back before being asked to execute the manoeuvre. It is important that the horse is positioned so that it has room to carry out the movement.

Finish the lesson off in rising trot, encouraging the horse to stretch down, and then ask the rider to dismount on the offside and then remount from the same side. The rider can then walk on a long rein to let the horse cool down and allow her to clear up any areas that she is anxious about. Finally, wish her luck and show an interest in the result of the test, whether it is positive or negative.

Adult working at Medium dressage level

Mother and daughter share a nine-year-old Medium level dressage pony; today's 45 minute lesson is with mother. The pony has had a respiratory problem and care must be taken not to overstress it. The aim of the lesson is to improve the collection in canter, as the previous dressage test sheets have shown this to be a weakness.

The rider is a logical learner and likes to understand thoroughly what she is being asked to achieve. She is a regular client so instructor and pupil are well bonded and already have a clearly defined approach to warming up. This includes a substantial amount of walking, bending and stretching the pony to establish flexibility and acceptance of the rein. This is followed by rising trot and canter on both reins, including circles and squares. Once pony and rider are warmed up the instructor can work on the canter to try to achieve the aim of the lesson. Working on a large circle the rider is asked to go forwards to working canter, then collect the canter for a few steps before moving the canter on again. The instructor observes the pony and when it lowers its quarters tells the rider that this has happened in order to develop the rider's 'feel'. Depending on the progress made the instructor may then introduce 10 m circles in collected canter, within the 20 m circle, suggesting corrections to the pony and rider throughout. The pony is then brought back to walk and the work evaluated by the rider and the instructor. The instructor then checks that the rider is happy to progress.

Some lateral work in walk gives the pony time to recover from the canter work, bearing in mind that he has had a respiratory problem, before moving on to half-pass in canter. The exercise is worked from the three-quarter line across the arena for as long as the pony feels comfortable and balanced. It may be that the rider finds this movement quite difficult in which case it may be useful for the instructor to get on the pony and demonstrate. This enables the rider to see what is required and the pony benefits from the extra expertise of the trainer.

After the instructor has ridden, the pony may seem quite tired, in which case the rider may decide not to remount and try again; however, this option is always open. The pony is walked to cool it off while the work is discussed and plans for the following week are made.

It is vital not to expect the pupil to do everything in one lesson. Plan strategically and be pleased with even the least progress.

The class flat lesson

The general objectives of a lesson on the flat are twofold:

- to stimulate the rider's interest in the horse's way of going;
- for the rider to maintain a good position throughout.

In this case the lesson is for riding club amateur riders competing at Novice dressage and the aims are:

- to accentuate the rider's feel of the correct sequence of footfalls at all paces;
- to move up and down the gears within the pace.

The lesson is taking place in an indoor school from 7–8 PM. The ride consists of six men and women of mixed ability and experience. The horses probably will have travelled to the venue and range in type from a pony to a heavyweight hunter, and in age from 4 to 18 years of age. The horses will be equipped with a variety of tack and will be very precious to their owners, they are their 'children' and the riders will want constructive comment not criticism.

Follow the rules we have previously discussed:

- Get to know your ride.
- If you cannot remember names, write them down.
- Agree the goals for today.
- Ensure the goals are clearly identifiable to the riders.
- 'Feel' and its development is always relevant.

Implement the lesson plan in five stages as follows.

Warm up

Allow the riders and horses to warm up on both reins in their own way. This gives you time to assess them and their horses' way of going. Look at:

- rider position;
- rider influence;
- the horses' paces;
- suppleness;
- balance;
- acceptance of the aids;
- empathy between horse and rider;
- empathy between rider and teacher.

Try to give each horse and rider an equal amount of attention. This may not be possible if a 'safety situation' arises, in other words one rider may need more help in order to avoid a hazardous situation arising. It is a good idea to work from either the front or the rear of the ride when making corrections. If the ride is in open order keep a careful mental note of to whom your comments have been addressed.

Walk

After the warm up check that the riders are all happy with their horses and their tack and ask them if they have warmed up as normal. Move on to explain the next exercise, for example, ask them to make a transition from free walk on a long rein to medium walk. Ask them how it feels. Are the steps equal? Is the horse accepting the bit? Is the horse 'in front of the leg'? You may not ask each question to each rider; instead spread the questions out to keep everybody involved.

Trot

In either rising or sitting trot – you will have to experiment to see which suits each rider best – work towards lengthening the stride. It is often difficult for inexperienced riders to feel lengthening so you could ask them to count the number of strides taken from quarter marker to quarter marker. Ask if the number of strides taken changed. Did the horse stay in balance? Is he still accepting the bit?

Canter

Ask each rider to canter on a circle while the other members of the ride circle at the other end of the school or stand and watch. Cones can help to keep the circle true and counting can help the rider monitor the regularity of the rhythm or assess lengthening of stride. Encourage feedback from the observers as well as the rider to train them to be observant and to keep them involved throughout.

Debrief and cool down
While the horses and riders are cooling down they can be debriefed.
Ask them what they felt was the greatest benefit to either themselves
or their horses. Give them some advice and work to do at home.

Jumping lessons

The young horse

Lesson one
The aim of the lesson is to introduce the young horse to jumping with
a rider. The horse should be warmed up in walk, trot and canter using
large circles, changes of rein and simple transitions. The warm up
period should last a minimum of 15 minutes, including some breaks.
The rider should be encouraged to have his/her stirrups at jumping
length throughout. The rider and trainer then establish, through
discussion, how the horse has responded during the warm up period.
Assuming that the horse has been previously worked over trotting
poles, this exercise can be used to promote the horse's concentration
and agility. The trainer can then assess the horse over a cross pole to
ascertain:

- the horse's attitude;
- technique;
- natural talent and athleticism;
- the rider's position and influence.

On the basis of this assessment, introduce a placing pole (Fig. 6.6) if it
will help:

- improve the take-off platform;
- increase the horse's concentration;
- improve athleticism;
- steady an impetuous horse;
- steady an impetuous rider.

The placing pole is usually laid about 8 ft (2.4 m) in front of the fence;
this distance should be carefully monitored and adjusted where
necessary. If a group of horses is working together the pole has to be

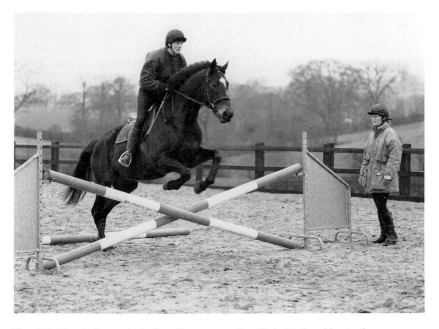

Fig. 6.6 A placing pole before the cross pole will help the rider to become more aware of rhythm and distance.

set at a distance that is compatible for the whole group. If the horse tries to take off before the pole, consider moving the pole out to 16–18 ft (4.9–5.5 m), one canter stride before the fence, or having a series of poles 4 ft 6 in (1.4 m) apart with the last one 8 ft (2.4 m) from the fence. Work the horse over this, in both directions. Then move on to a vertical fence with a clear groundline on both sides. This may take up most of lesson one, as time must be allowed for the horse to cool down and stretch. Feedback from the rider is necessary in order to agree the homework and the goals for next week's lesson.

Lesson two
The aim of the second lesson is to introduce the young horse to jumping a spread fence (Fig. 6.7). This is usually an ascending oxer with the lower part either a cross or simply a horizontal rail. There must be a clearly defined groundline. Warm up the horse and rider using lesson one as a template. When the horse is ready, introduce the spread, either from trot or by introducing a second fence 45 ft (13.7 m) away from the small vertical. This will allow the horse three easy strides. If using this second method leave the back pole off the spread

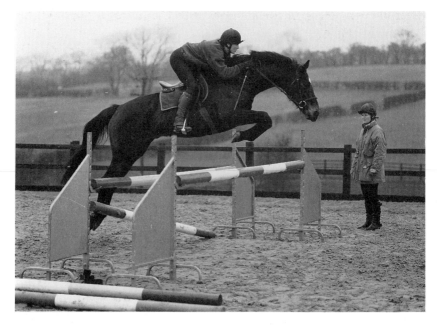

Fig. 6.7   This rider's position is enabling the young horse to jump a spread fence with confidence.

fence the first time the horse jumps it so that you can check the distance. Also check the key factors as before:

- the horse's attitude;
- technique;
- natural talent and athleticism;
- the rider's position and influence.

Always confirm with the rider that your observations and what he/she feels are complementary to each other. This ensures accurate assessment of the present situation and allows suitable plans to be made for the future.

Young horses can be jumped two or three times a week provided that the going is good and that the sessions are not prolonged; 30–40 minutes from start to finish is adequate.

The class jumping lesson

Grid work – novice horses
The aim of the lesson is to improve the horse's agility and balance. The class has riders and horses of mixed ability and experience but they are

generally competing at novice level with the fences around 3 ft 5 in (1.06 m) in height.

The grid (e.g. Fig. 6.8) should be set up prior to the lesson. The fences should start at about 2 ft 6 in (0.7 m) high and build up to 3 ft 5 in (1.06 m). In a grid the parallels can be square and about 3 ft 3 in (1 m) wide initially.

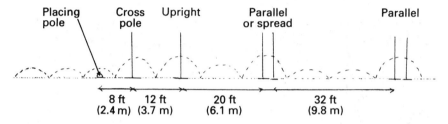

Fig. 6.8   Grid work – novice horses.

The class should be warmed up using all paces and circles, changes of direction and transitions. Check the riders' ability to maintain a balanced seat both in trot and canter. Their stirrups should be short enough for this to be effective. Throughout the warm up discuss the exercises so that the riders are satisfied and know where they are going. Make sure that all the riders receive an equal share of comment and help.

Prior to working down the grid, warm up over a single fence with a placing pole and then introduce the grid with one component at a time. Most of the work is done in trot. Ideally build the grid so that it can be jumped off both reins. If this is not possible, then make a note of which rein has been used this time so that there can be a change on the next occasion.

Throughout the lesson use the following critical assessment guidelines to ensure that all aspects are covered:

- the attitude of the horse – confidence, calmness and enthusiasm;
- the technique and athleticism of the horse;
- the balance and rhythm down the grid and on the approach and landing;
- the rider's balance and influence.

As with all exercises, adjust the heights, distances and nature of the fence to reflect the current needs of the horses in the group. Remember to allow sufficient time for debrief and feedback. Finally, agree future goals and the strategies that are to be used to achieve them.

Grid work – advanced horses
The aim of the lesson is to develop the horse's rhythm and technique. The horses warm up as before but the emphasis is on canter work, including transitions within the pace and flying changes. Simple lateral work and rein back can also be introduced. Encourage the riders to liken their horses to ballerinas who must warm up all of their muscles prior to performance. Muscles that are warm have a good supply of blood and are thus less prone to damage.

Again the grid (e.g. Fig. 6.9) should be constructed before the lesson. The fences can be up to 3 ft 7 in (1.09 m) high and 4 ft 6 in (1.4 m) wide. Poles can be used between the fences to regulate the stride – use the following distances as a guide: 12 ft (3.7 m) on the landing side of the fence and 8–9 ft (2.4–2.7 m) before the next fence. It is vital during this sort of work to pay great attention to the horse's footfalls so that the poles or fences can be adjusted as necessary.

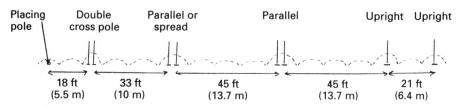

Fig. 6.9 Grid work – advanced horses.

If riders are unfamiliar with canter poles, these can be practised separately from the gridwork, the usual distance between the poles being 9 ft (2.7 m) for the average horse. Long grids such as the one illustrated in Fig. 6.9 can only be used where there is sufficient room for the horse to approach the grid in a balanced canter and to be able to land and flow through the turn after the grid.

During all class work riders should be encouraged to keep on the move so that the horses do not become cold and stiff through standing around. Strict discipline must be enforced when the grid is being jumped:

- No following close on another horse's heels.
- Ensure free access to the grid.
- Ensure riders are aware of other riders jumping out of the grid.

It is essential that the jumping trainer is confident in his/her ability to measure distances with a fair degree of accuracy. Develop this skill by striding a distance, say 9 ft (3 m), and then measuring it with a tape. Do this for longer distances until you can keep a regular, even and accurate stride length. Check your distances a couple of times a year to maintain accuracy; while a couple of centimetres is not crucial, 1 ft (0.03 m) is significant. When measuring distances remember to measure from the final element to the first element of an obstacle, except in the case of a hog's-back type fence or a bank when eventing.

Advanced individual show jumping lesson

The long term aim is to jump a clear round at Badminton. The short term aim is to jump clear at the next competition. The problem is that the horse is inclined to become quick and then gain too much ground through the combination fences. Added to this the rider is inclined to 'fire' the horse at a fence (Fig. 6.10).

In this scenario the rider and trainer have worked together previously. Work the horse in with the emphasis on keeping him calm, use

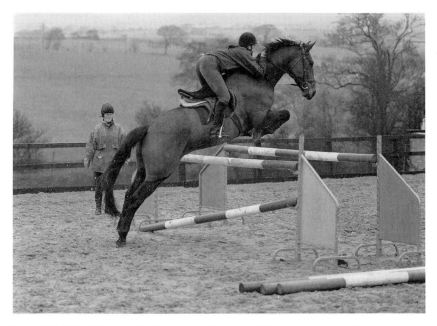

Fig. 6.10 This rider is a little 'in front of the horse' thus encouraging him to make up too much ground through the combination fence.

transitions, both from pace to pace and within the pace. Jumping is introduced over a cross pole and placing pole with the cross 3 ft 3 in (1 m) high in the centre (Fig. 6.11).

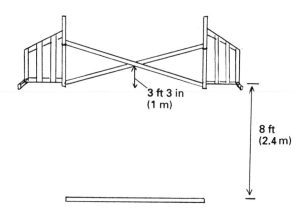

Fig. 6.11 Cross pole and placing pole.

The horse should be worked over this on both reins from trot, but allowing canter at the pole. Counteract any inclination by the horse to rush the fence by asking the rider to circle the horse away or to walk a few steps before returning to trot. The cross pole can then be made into a vertical 3 ft 3 in (1 m) high, and then a parallel 3 ft 3 in (1 m) square, which are still jumped from trot with a placing pole. The emphasis should be on rhythm, and while transitions can be used the horse should not be stifled on the approach to the fence. The rider must avoid moving the upper body excessively and should be encouraged to find a balanced seat. Make sure that you also comment on the horse's technique so that you help the rider develop feel.

If the horse is inclined to rush on landing, use a pole on the landing side of the fence, 12 ft (3.7 m) away from the fence. A plank can also be used, it will not roll and it gives the horse more to focus on.

Move on to jumping in canter, starting with a vertical at 3 ft 3 in (1 m) and raising it to 3 ft 5 in (1.06 m). Agree with the rider whether to keep the placing pole at 8 ft (2.4 m) or to move it out to 18 ft (5.5 m), allowing room for a stride before take-off. Introduce a second vertical about 3 ft 5 in (1.06 m) high, 21 ft (6.4 m) away (Fig. 6.12). If the horse jumps too big and too quickly going into the double, put down a pole between the two elements to regulate the stride (Fig. 6.13). Add a third element to make a combination. Start with this 30 ft (9 m) from the

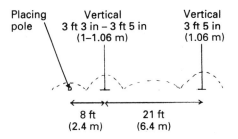

Fig. 6.12

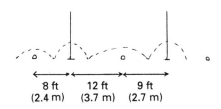

Fig. 6.13

second vertical until both the trainer and rider have evaluated the horse's response. Canter poles can be used if necessary (Fig. 6.14).

If the last element is a parallel 3 ft 7 in (1.09 m) square this will help to back the horse off the fences and allow him to use his body and legs more effectively. The rider must be encouraged to sit as still as possible and to feel the strides. Even advanced riders will find it beneficial to count the strides as it will help stop them anticipating the jump. Gradually this exercise can be built up to a maximum height of 3 ft 11 in (1.2 m), but keep the distances short. The placing pole can be removed from in front of the first fence, but care must be taken that the rider does not over-ride the fence.

The trainer must always be on the look out for any need to adjust the exercise should it cease to be beneficial. At all times the rider's position, balance and influence must be checked and corrected if

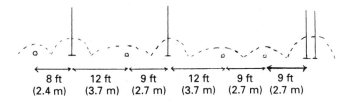

Fig. 6.14

necessary. Often with such exercises it has to be explained to the rider that the benefits may not be immediate. It may take many sessions using a wide variety of exercises before the horse begins to think for himself. If after several sessions there is no improvement, a further evaluation may be necessary to try to identify if there is a more obscure reason for the horse being impetuous. It is often valuable for the trainer to see the horse and rider at a competition; they may both react differently under stress. Video is useful but can sometimes be rather flattering.

At the end of the session remember to cool the horse down slowly and to keep the horse on the move during feedback sessions. Set homework and discuss the working in pattern at a competition and agree any changes that may be needed.

Cross country schooling

The novice horse or rider
The aim is to build confidence and establish correct techniques. It is preferable not to have a novice horse *and* rider partnership.

Building confidence Building confidence is achieved by slowly increasing the severity of the test in each lesson. Inevitably there will be times when either the horse or the rider is unsure; discuss the fear with the rider and explain why it will be a positive move to try to overcome that fear. For example, an inexperienced child has fallen off a couple of times down a drop fence. She comes to you, at her mother's insistence, in order to learn not to fall off under normal circumstances. First of all watch the child negotiate a very small simple drop fence, for example a log on a slope, not under trees, on difficult terrain or into water. You notice that the child has two main problems:

(1) She is afraid and in consequence does not kick the pony into the fence, so he jumps awkwardly and gives her an uncomfortable jump.
(2) Her legs slide back, she becomes unstable and lands around the pony's ears.

The teacher has to take these two problems and tackle them side by side, giving slight priority to getting the rider to move the pony into the fence with more confidence and authority. This is accomplished by working them over a straightforward fence on the flat or up a slight slope. The fence should be a log, a brush fence or a simple ascending spread. As the combination becomes more confident (Fig. 6.15) the teacher can correct the leg position and try to establish some feedback from the pupil so that she can tell the teacher when she begins to feel more secure. From here the combination can be taken back to the small drop fence and the same techniques applied.

- Don't try to solve the problem all in one go.
- Do stop when you are pleased with the progress.
- Don't let yourself be coerced by the parent to go on beyond the moment that you have identified as being the best time to stop.
- Do use good schooling grounds.
- Don't use inadequate, flimsy and narrow fences. It is always worth paying a bit more for good facilities.

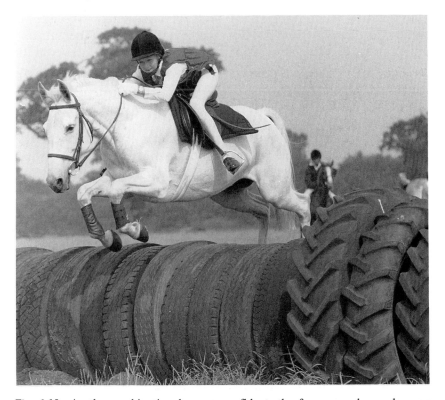

Fig. 6.15 As the combination become confident, the fences can be made more challenging.

A horse that lacks confidence is more difficult as you cannot discuss the problem with him! A young or inexperienced horse that lacks confidence needs a confident, but not bullying, rider. Before he jumps solid cross country fences he must be confident and well schooled over show jumps, so that his technique is reasonably well established. The rider and trainer should also know his degree of ability so that they can keep the questions that are asked at a suitable level. Assuming that the horse is a four or five year old and a novice jumper, there are a number of options open. The next step may be to school him over cross country fences in the company of a more experienced horse which can give the young horse a lead. Some riders and trainers advocate hunting. How beneficial this will be depends on:

- the type of country that is hunted over;
- the size of the 'field' i.e. the number of people;
- the temperament of the horse.

If the horse is naturally keen and forward-going, hunting can exacerbate the situation. Horses that are calm and rather uncommitted in their approach to jumping often draw confidence from the experience of splashing through puddles, jumping small ditches, hedges and rails. However, the rider must have great self discipline so that he/she does not get carried away and ask too much of the young horse.

Another option is novice team chasing. Again there are advantages and disadvantages. If you can choose a team that is prepared to school over the course for the benefit of your horse that is one thing. However, if the team is out to win, the competition may do the young horse more harm than good.

All these means of building confidence are only part of the whole picture. At the end of the day the horse has to be able to perform alone; schooling sessions that introduce and build on this are therefore essential. Never allow a client to take a horse to a cross country competition if it has not been schooled cross country. It is asking for a disaster to happen.

Establishing technique   What sort of technique does the cross country horse need? The key is establishing rhythm and balance. Each horse will have his own technique over a fence. Excessive basculing over cross country fences is not desirable as it slows the horse down and can unbalance the horse when landing down steep drops or into water.

The rider's technique must ensure that he/she is able to maintain his/her own balance to complement that of the horse.

The rider's technique can be improved by simply cantering over varying terrain and keeping balance. Experiment by altering the length of the stirrups and asking the rider to feedback to you when he/she feels comfortable. Remember, the rider's comfort must not be at the expense of the horse.

Next move the horse 'up and down the gears,' i.e. through canter and gallop, utilizing any hills and varying terrain that is available. This is to allow the rider to find out how to adjust his/her body weight to give maximum confidence, security and effectiveness. Whenever possible novice riders should have schoolmaster horses and ponies so that they can establish the best possible technique. Once they are secure and confident the riders can attempt simple cross country fences. The teacher has to encourage balance, rhythm and the correct tempo for the situation in hand.

Never:

- force a rider to jump something he/she is really afraid of;
- make a rider go faster than he/she is confident to manage;
- ridicule a rider – remember your fears (spiders, heights or snakes); that is what the frightened rider is feeling.

Always finish on a high note, preferably when horse and rider are keen to continue. It is said of a good meal 'stop while you are wanting more'; training horses and riders is rather similar!

Advanced cross country schooling
The aims of advanced cross country schooling are varied and may include:

- solving a problem;
- getting to know a new horse;
- progressing from one level to another, for example from Intermediate to Advanced.

The most common reason for schooling the more advanced horses cross country is to solve a problem. For this scenario we have a horse that has fallen jumping into water at Gatcombe. Two important factors are that the horse is aimed for Blenheim and that it has not been taken through the grades by the present rider, so its schooling history is difficult to establish accurately.

We must first try to establish why the horse fell by using video recordings and the observations of expert onlookers, as well as the feel from the rider. In this case it is established that the horse tends to 'back off' when approaching water. This is not unusual but it does tend to encourage the rider to over-ride the fence. The horse was also felt to have left his back legs on the fence, thus tipping him onto his head as he landed in the water. However, the rider, who is highly competent, is confident in the horse despite the fall.

With these two problems in mind the horse is taken to a cross country schooling ground with a water complex which has a variety of routes into the water, differing in severity from novice to advanced. The water has a firm base, is not too deep and the take-off before the jump is reinforced to minimize slipping.

The first priority is to try to generate greater confidence in the horse by schooling him over some easy water obstacles, after which he can progress to more demanding tests. The horse must not be galloped at the water; this will only unnerve him further. He must jump into the water because he feels safe to do so and because he wants to please the rider. Remember that the bitting and fit of the tack must not itself cause the horse a problem.

Initially the horse must be warmed up and jumped over some straightforward fences, including some simple drop fences (Fig. 6.16). His responses on the approach to the fence should be monitored and reported back to the trainer. It is essential that the trainer is able to see the key fences, the drop and water fences. Cross country trainers should invest in some good binoculars and possibly some portable loudspeaker equipment or ear phones for the rider to facilitate communication. Feedback throughout the session is necessary so that the trainer can make suggestions that will lead to improved performance.

If schooling fails to encourage the older horse to be more positive a compromise may have to be reached. Provided that the 'backing off' does not result in a refusal, or leave him so short of impulsion that he cannot jump the fence, the rider will have to take this behaviour into consideration when walking water fences at a competition. Whenever complex or large fences have to be jumped there is often an alternative route. Bearing the horse's attitude in mind, it is well to consider the alternative route at water complexes when establishing the competition strategy.

The second aspect to be considered is that the horse left his hind legs

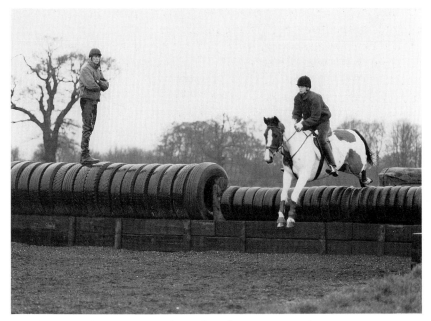

Fig. 6.16 Warming up over a simple drop fence.

on the fence. This is quite common in experienced horses jumping down drops, and usually jumping into water is a similar experience as the water is frequently at a lower level than the take-off. Schooling over simple fences into water, such as a log, helps encourage the horse to jump out as far as possible. More importantly, check the rider's balance; the upper body must not collapse over the horse's neck on landing, and the lower leg must be secure with a deep heel. If the rider is unbalanced a simple mistake can dislodge the rider and thus shake the horse's confidence.

Never:

● chase the horse over the fence with whips or use other forceful means. If this sort of coercion is necessary the question must be asked 'is this horse suited for the job in hand?';
● school over water fences that have insecure footing.

Always be satisfied with a little progress. Remember your objective ruler; if you progress from 5.5 to 6 out of ten, you have achieved a short term goal!

Part II
Specialist Teaching and Coaching

7 Teaching Children

Teaching children can be a rich and satisfying experience. It is also a tremendous responsibility. These are the riders of the future and the attitudes that they learn from you can affect every aspect of their lives. You can help give them confidence or you can undermine what confidence they have.

Before looking at any special techniques that teaching children may involve, perhaps we should define what is meant by children. I would suggest that, in this context, we are considering those in the age range 6 to 15. As we are all aware, children appear to mature much earlier today, and at which point they gradually become young adults will be quite variable.

The qualities needed for teaching children are obviously similar to those required for teaching adults, but most children require the learning to be an enjoyable experience. Being in school can be stressful and academic learning is not 'fun' for the majority of children. These factors are of major importance when developing a successful technique for teaching children to ride. There is also a clear division between the children who have their own ponies and those who do not and usually ride in a riding school.

What makes a child want to learn to ride? For some the love of ponies seems to be born into them. These children may not necessarily come from a horsey background, but simply love the touch, smell and general ambience that ponies emanate. These children are usually highly motivated. There are others whose families own horses, they grow up with them and riding is as normal as playing football or swimming. Their peers also ride, it is socially acceptable and, through the Pony Club, fun (Fig. 7.1). Many of these children ride when young but later drift away into other chosen activities.

Children with ambitious parents, regardless of whether or not they own ponies, are arguably the most difficult to deal with. Equally, the child whose parents wish him/her to ride because it is the 'done thing'

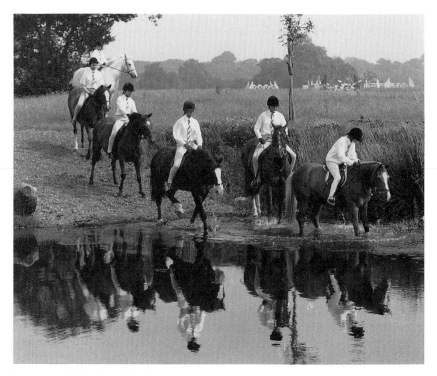

Fig. 7.1   Riding should be fun.

are often unwilling pupils. Children with special needs are dealt with elsewhere but they are usually particularly rewarding, as their gains from this activity extend beyond merely learning to ride.

The Pony Club mostly caters for children with their own ponies, although in a few areas there are branches based at riding schools designed for the non-pony owner. Although Pony Clubs were originally attached to Hunts, there are increasing numbers of branches that are area-based. Some branches are so large that they are divided into areas within the branch.

The Pony Club Instructor's Handbook gives very good guidelines on the procedures expected at rallies and how to go about teaching different standards of rides. The Pony Club runs instructor courses both nationally and locally, but at present it is not mandatory to have a qualification.

The main difficulty for the Pony Club instructor is that quite often the lesson is a 'one-off'. You may have a group of children for half a day, or maybe a whole day, you may not know the children and be given little direction by the District Commissioner or Rally Organizer.

Try to identify a plan and agree a goal with all those involved, for example the parent, organizer, child and possibly even the child's regular instructor. This can be quite difficult but it is even more important than usual to try to do this. Allow sufficient time to find out the children's names – write them down if you find it difficult to remember names. Ask about their ponies and find out what the combination have done together; at the same time check the tack for safety and fit. All this is very worthwhile and gives you the information necessary to be able to plan your lesson. If you have very small children, say four to seven year olds, some may need to be on the leading rein. This adds an extra tricky dimension to the lesson. Who is in charge – you or the pony leader? Try to reach an amicable arrangement about this from the outset.

Right at the beginning it is very important that you try to assess the children's confidence. This may be quite apparent in the early introduction, but, if not, further clues should emerge during the assessment period. The purpose of the assessment is to try to check that the children's statements of competence are reasonably accurate – they can do what they say they can do. If their confidence or competence is not as expected this assessment will allow you to adjust your lesson plan as necessary.

Any plan that you formulate must, of course, reflect the need to be highly safety-conscious at all times. This may hinder the speed of progress, but remember that if you ever have to ask yourself 'is this safe enough?', then the likelihood is that it is not safe enough. It is extremely difficult, perhaps impossible, to lay down or even suggest precise safety parameters; the judgement of the instructor is of paramount importance in all procedures. Of course there may be specific branch rules and this makes life easier for you as some of the responsibility has been removed. The best way to maintain a safe lesson is to be:

- vigilant;
- quick to spot any external distractions;
- quick to react if a child is becoming agitated, tired or even bored;
- quick to assess if a pony is starting to become disobedient or to act out of character.

If you have the children for a whole morning or afternoon, break the riding into manageable chunks, allow time for questions and encourage group discussion, even with small children. The purpose is to try to instil trust and confidence in you as the teacher, so that the children feel that they can talk to you. If when you ask a question there is little or no response, try to reword the question to enable an answer to be forthcoming. Do not terrorize the child if he clearly does not know what you are talking about.

Those of us privileged to teach children have a unique opportunity; the habits taught to the young are often there for life, so try to encourage good practice, enable learning and understanding to take place but do not take away the fun element. Remember above all:

'I hear and forget
I see and remember
I do and understand.'

If a demonstration is part of your lesson, try to break this down to show a step at a time. It can help to think of this in the following words: I do it normally, you watch carefully; I do it slow, now off you go.

One of the main problems that can occur with any lesson, but particularly with children who own their own ponies, is the difficult pony that disrupts the whole lesson. What can the instructor do? If the problem cannot be solved by adjusting the exercises given, then try to get some extra assistance; the assistant instructor can either lead the pony or take the combination away for a session on their own to try to sort out the problem. With older children it may be possible to suggest a work plan that they can carry out on their own before returning to the ride. Never focus all your attention on the one child and neglect the others. As far as possible equal attention should be paid to all the children in a ride. This takes a lot of practice and self discipline; one way to improve your technique in this area is to work your way from the front to the back of the ride and give a comment to each child. Do not worry if you cannot see something to correct quickly, instead give some praise or encouragement. It is important that when you make a correction, to the rider's position or the pony's way of going, you are able to give a reason why an adjustment should be made. You need not do this every time, but it can encourage the riders to try to comply with your requests if they can see a reason why they should. Also, because they understand, the improvement is more likely to be permanent.

Equipment may be limited at rallies, especially when teaching jumping. It is your responsibility to make the best use of what is available so that your ride has fun and progresses. For example, what sort of exercises could be beneficial if you were working the ride over trotting poles?

- Assuming that we are preparing to jump, shorten stirrups.
- Check the rider's ability to rise, sit and keep 'poised' position in open order around the poles.
- Carry out the same exercise and ask each child which position feels best and why.
- Count the rhythm towards the poles to encourage the children to evaluate the rhythm and adjust the tempo if necessary.
- Encourage the children to close their eyes on the approach and to keep counting the rhythm and to stay in balance.
- If blocks or similar equipment are available, raise alternate ends of the poles.
- Vary the distance between all the poles to give the children the feel of larger or smaller strides.
- Vary the rein contact – long and low to encourage stretching;
  - on a contact to improve impulsion;
  - on a loose rein to encourage attentiveness and to help develop balance.

It is an excellent idea to try to develop these plans for all types of lesson; by using your imagination you will develop your own lessons and make them interesting and demanding at an appropriate level for the participants.

The child learning in a riding school has some advantages and disadvantages. The advantages include the fact that the ponies are specially selected to suit the size, experience and aspirations of the riders. The environment is usually conducive to learning, for example there may be an enclosed arena, the instructors know the ponies and the equipment, which allows them to plan ahead with a greater degree of certainty that the plan can be carried out and that further progressive plans can follow over a series of lessons.

The main disadvantage of the child learning to ride at a riding school is the lack of opportunity to practise regularly. It is rarely practical to allow the same child to ride the same pony each time; bonding between pony and child is thus rare. Also, if the child is competitive, the opportunities to compete regularly are not normally readily available.

Physical development

Parents often ask the age at which children should start to learn to ride. The answer depends on what we mean by 'learn'. We know that by the time a child is four years old, 50% of his/her intelligence is developed, an additional 30% develops between the ages of four and eight and the remaining 20% by the time the young adult is 17. The skill of riding is a dual one; one part being physical control of the body, the other being the ability to respond to teaching in order to ride the pony effectively. On the whole, children below the age of seven, riding once a week, find it difficult to progress. So, for children between the ages of four and seven, riding tends to be a pleasurable experience, but not one in which progressive learning has to take place. The other factor to consider is the lack of physical development at this age; the child's ability to influence the pony is therefore limited. Young children have relatively large heads and short legs which affects their balance.

The very young probably benefit most by simply sitting on the pony, being made comfortable by being shown how to sit and hold the reins and then being allowed to experience the feeling of sitting on the pony in walk. They are being given the opportunity to experience riding. The slightly older child may be able to cope with an explanation first and then carrying out the chosen practical activity.

Often the selection of suitable ponies in the riding school situation is out of the control of the individual instructor, but, as far as possible, the ponies should enable both the teacher and the child to progress as correctly as possible, so that excessive kicking or pulling on the reins is discouraged.

Most children are instinctively competitive and this should be borne in mind and used as an aid to learning. The instructor can organize games or competitions within the group or simple tests with rewards for achieving targets. This acts as a stimulus for both teacher and pupil; combined enjoyment and performance are likely to enhance the learning outcomes.

Specialist coaching

Even at this early stage there are instructors who specialize in various aspects of teaching children. You may, as an instructor, have a special interest in one area and would like to become involved, for example, in training children for the show ring or show jumping (Fig. 7.2). Once you have done your initial training and attained basic qualifications, for example the British Horse Society Assistant Instructors' examination, it is wise to apprentice yourself to an established trainer in your chosen sphere. The special skills needed to present a pony in the show ring or to compete in top level pony show jumping need to be developed. If you are not exposed to the specialist discipline on a regular basis you will not develop the necessary skills of observation, nor will you be aware of the psychological pressure put on a child who wants to win, whether for his/her own needs or to satisfy the expectations of others.

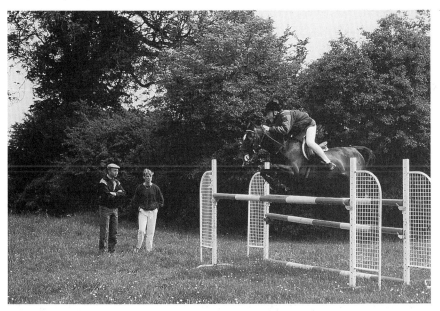

Fig. 7.2   The trainer may specialize in teaching show jumping. (*Courtesy:* Elizabeth Furth)

A suggested children's coaching code

- Be reasonable in your demands of young riders' time, energy and enthusiasm. Remember, they have other interests.
- Teach your rider that the rules of the game are mutual agreements which no one should evade or break. This is particularly so where the welfare of the horse is involved.
- Avoid overtraining talented riders. 'Average' riders need and deserve equal time.

- Remember that children ride for fun and enjoyment and that winning is only part of the picture. Never ridicule or yell at children for making mistakes or losing a competition.
- The length and schedule of training and competitions should take into account the child's level of maturity.
- Develop respect for the ability of opponents as well as for the judges' assessment and that of other trainers and instructors.
- Follow the advice of a doctor in determining when an injured rider should be ready to ride again.
- Remember that children need a coach they can respect. Be generous in your praise and set a good example.

Competitive children must be encouraged to evaluate their performance positively, whether they are winners or not, so that the goals are set on outcomes rather than performance success. One of the difficulties of our sport is that the outcome of a competition may be dictated by a purely subjective judgement. This subjectivity is based on certain expectations and if the child is not aware of these expectations he/she can be disappointed and upset with the result. Therefore coaches must make themselves thoroughly familiar with the expectations, rules and protocol of the discipline they are involved with.

The coach can encourage children, even at an early age, to think in terms of personal bests. Obviously in our sport 'personal' is a joint term for both pony and child. Success is measured in terms of effort, improvement and personal bests, not just winning. These three targets are aspects that children have some control over and concentrating on these helps to build their self motivation and to develop a positive attitude to competition.

As in all teaching the coach must have a positive attitude using praise and encouragement and avoiding insults and humiliation. Certainly punishment must be avoided at all costs. These points are even more crucial when teaching children than in any other sphere. On the other hand the coach must be careful not to push the gifted child too hard in order to bask in the reflected glory. As has been the case with some young tennis players, precocious talent can be quickly burned out before the young person has really learned to live. Even for the keenest competitor there must be a life outside their chosen sport.

It is of positive value that children have heros or role models on which to base their own techniques and aspirations. It is valuable to the coach if they are aware of this and use the knowledge to develop confidence and ambition. This development can act as a basis for regular positive feedback. Your encouragement will help them to begin to trust their own judgement rather than to respond to peer or parent pressure.

Up to the age of 12, most young children think that by trying harder they will improve. Certainly some effort is essential, but if the child is working hard and not improving on his/her 'personal best', the coach should try to evaluate why there is no improvement. The coach can then either set about solving the problem or help the child and parent to accept the limitations that exist. There are a variety of routes for the coach to explore, for example the pony may be of limited ability; this may be rectified by changing the goal or changing the pony.

The child may be afraid of going cross country. Try to find out the basis of this fear. If the child is physically afraid of falling off and being hurt, this fear may never be overcome and it may be better to channel the child's energies in a different direction, dressage perhaps. We must never forget that the child who is not enjoying his/her sport is not going to be a winner and may even give up the sport entirely if pressured.

Everyone learns in a different way. Because of this a change in trainer is sometimes beneficial. The child may not hit it off with a certain style of teaching while a different teacher may suit him/her better. However, frequent changes of trainer should not be encouraged as it takes time to form a bond between child and trainer and the varying philosophies and techniques can prove muddling for the young rider.

Do not allow your young pupils to expect perfection; striving for perfection has a place, but it is far better to aim to do your best and seek tangible targets rather than ultimate perfection.

There are some overall aspects to keep in mind when teaching children:

- Keep the lesson and your attitude positive.
- Look for things to praise, especially for those who are not high flyers.
- Praise good behaviour, particularly relationships with other children and accepting the judge's decision. Other examples may be good behaviour when unable to ride the pony they had hoped for or not being able to take part in an activity they had looked forward to.
- Praise effort and good performance more than results, for example a stylish good round that was not quick enough to win.

- When a mistake follows a good movement, do not forget to praise the good part.
- Do not mix praise and criticism; it is confusing, for example 'Good approach, pity about the landing'.

Another important overall aspect of teaching children is dealing with mistakes or poor performance. Trainer, pupil and parent have to accept that mistakes are a valuable source of learning. This is why the trainer should not always take over to protect the child from making mistakes, unless safety is an issue. It is more valuable to encourage children to work out for themselves what went wrong. For example, pony and rider have an uncomfortable jump; the instructor could ask, 'What do you think caused this?'; the answer may be, 'Not enough impulsion'. The instructor can now take this further to test understanding with the question, 'Where?'; answer, 'Through the turn'. As the child has shown good understanding, it is more likely that when the exercise is repeated the problem will be remedied. Many teachers do not allow the students to find out for themselves what went wrong, so problem solving is always left to the teacher. This does not equip the riders to cope when they are left on their own. Obviously the child needs to have reached a certain stage of maturity, probably ten years old and upwards, before simple self evaluation can take place.

Riders do not mean to make mistakes so do not use hostility and sarcasm as a means of correction or reprimand.

The age at which children start to ride will influence their physical ability. The child's physical development as he/she gets older will affect the way that you teach. A child's constantly changing physique will, and should, limit your goals. For example, the child may simply be unable to maintain the pony in the balance and rhythm required for success. We often see a child riding beautifully at 12 years of age, but then a growth spurt and puberty upset the picture and it can take quite some time for the child to regain his/her original performance, indeed some never do. Most of this change is due to the fact that just before the adolescent growth spurt a child's arms and legs are disproportionately long; this will affect co-ordination and balance and an unbalanced rider leads to an unbalanced horse.

Children differ markedly at the same age; age itself has little to do with muscular or bodily strength and it is often inappropriate to group children by age. It is often better to look at the child's physical maturity, and, if appropriate, riding ability and any Pony Club tests that have been achieved. How children are grouped is a key factor in allowing the instructor to achieve progressive, influential instruction.

Puberty has a dynamic effect on children, both physically and mentally. Boys often become more assertive, they also become stronger which affects their stamina and means that they are less likely to tire. Girls often change their attitude to those around them; their peers, parents and instructors. This sometimes also extends to their attitude to their pony. As they come to terms with adulthood they may appear not to be as single-minded as they have been previously. Girls are often embarrassed by the changes in their bodies, they may try to hide this by becoming round shouldered, collapsing at the waist and tucking their bottoms underneath them. Of course this will not always happen, but it is important that the teacher is sensitive to the possibilities. At one time girls were told 'I must, I must, increase my bust' while they were riding to encourage better posture; current thinking is unlikely to endorse such adages.

Another factor to take into consideration is stamina. Children cannot ride actively for prolonged periods of time. Before adolescence children do not produce energy as efficiently as adults. The average six year old breathes in 38 litres of air to extract a litre of oxygen against the 28 litres needed by an 18 year old. This means that young children must work harder than adults to provide the energy their bodies need. Up to the age of about ten, boys and girls produce roughly the same amount of aerobic energy. During puberty their efficiency increases but girls generally stop improving around the age of 14 while boys continue to improve up to about 18 years of age.

During a normal riding lesson this may not be very significant, if the pony is well behaved and the child is at ease with the situation. However, prolonged activity such as cross-country or a lively pony out hunting may well significantly tire a child and limit his/her ability to perform.

In general, horse riders have never considered the need to be physically fit to compete, but we should really take just as much care as any other athlete. We care for the ponies and ensure that they are fit enough by giving them a sensible diet, access to water and a strategic exercise programme. Children who take riding seriously should also be encouraged to look after their bodies and to ensure that they give their mounts as much help as possible. Equally, encourage your young rider to understand the reasons why it is good for both horse and rider to warm up and cool down properly. This is another area where we riders are not as disciplined as we should be.

There is a wide range of equine activities for the young rider to choose from, from showing to three day eventing. It is outside the scope of this book to detail the requirements of each discipline, but the guidelines for teaching remain throughout and the following scenarios are designed to illustrate this.

We have a child who is keen to get into the European Pony three day event team. Normally a child with this ambition would have been competing successfully at Pony Club level and may already have a private trainer. What are the important aspects in this situation? In order to build up confidence the child must first have a clear understanding of the requirements of each phase of the test. Never just assume that because a child has been competing that he/she thoroughly understands what is required. Take time over each step. For example, the dressage test:

- Explain what the judge is looking for.
- Discuss the pony's strengths and weaknesses;
  - how are you going to capitalize on the strengths and improve the weak points?
  - If possible make use of video to monitor progress.
- Analyse test sheets, preferably with all the parties involved.
- Study arena craft by watching top riders perform.
- Discuss and decide on the 'what if' scenario;
  - what if he canters on the wrong leg?
  - what if he tenses up as he enters the arena?

This sort of mental rehearsal is an invaluable way of helping all competitors to cope when things do not go according to plan. All this work can be gone through at home prior to any warm up competitions, so that by the time a team trial takes place, established methods of preparation are well in place.

The amount of practice needed for any phase has to be tempered by the individual child and other commitments, such as school. The schooling of the pony must never turn into a chore or the fun element and hence the motivation are lost. Be aware that riding after school can be very stressful, especially around exam time, so do not expect high quality work at these times. Discuss with the child how he/she feels and what would be the most suitable training programme for that day or that week.

At competitions the emphasis must always be positive; if the pony is not going at his best when you arrive there, it is too late to do anything about it, so keep concentrating on the good aspects. Many riders, especially children, can arrive at a competition and actually expect their ponies to go better than they do at home – on the whole this is not realistic.

Children vary in the amount of back up they like to receive at a competition, but intensive coaching is rarely productive. In the dressage phase, for example, aim to get the pony going quietly and confidently through simple movements; remember we are trying to enhance his athletic ability, we do not want to make him tense and apprehensive by asking for a series of complicated exercises. Involve the child in assessing how the pony is going and decide together what else needs to be done. Try not to be distracted by how other ponies are going but keep focusing on your own rider's performance. It is almost always a good idea to watch a prior competitor's test to see how the arena is riding and how much time the judge is giving before the bell. The trainer needs to ensure that the riding-in phase is correctly timed and to check that the whole competition is running to schedule.

Whatever the outcome of the test, try to evaluate it as positively as possible; remember about personal bests and decide how you are going to measure this. Is it going to be by comparison with other riders that your pupil has competed against regularly? Using marks to evaluate the test is difficult unless the rider has ridden the same test for the same judge on a previous occasion. It might be that a particular movement is better, or indeed, the ultimate achievement – the pony and rider have competed to the best of their current ability.

Try not to make excuses for poor performance; the fact that a horse box drove by at the wrong moment, or that you arrived late and did not have enough time to warm up properly, needs to be addressed separately from your evaluation of the marks. Otherwise we can nearly always find an excuse for the performance not coming up to expectation without identifying the basic training weakness. Before discussing how a performance has gone, a child often needs time to unwind, so never jump down the child's throat the moment they have left the arena and say, 'Why didn't you kick here or pull there?'. Ideally let the child take the initiative and wait until he/she would like to discuss the outcome. Never let a child or adult take revenge on the pony if the performance has not been up to expectation.

At competitions where there is more than one phase or class, try to encourage your pupil to think about the next part as soon as possible. Be aware that if the child is nervous about any aspect of the competition, it is likely that other phases may suffer as a consequence. Above all, never let children feel that they cannot do something; make the task more simple if necessary. Try to avoid throwing them in at the deep end if they cannot swim!

You can appreciate from all this that the trainer's role is complex and diverse, but at the same time fascinating and rewarding.

Tips for teaching children

- Treat each child as an individual.
- Make sure they are ready to learn, emotionally as well as physically.
- Explain what you want, demonstrate and give plenty of time for them to practise.
- Keep practice and competition fun, varied and active.
- Let them use the skills in a meaningful situation as soon as possible.
- Correct mistakes one at a time.
- Start with simple skills before developing complex specialist skills.
- Listen to children, be on their wavelength, talk in their language and at their level.
- Be positive – encourage rather than criticize.
- Put the child's needs first, and winning second.
- Work with parents, not against them.
- Reinforce attitudes of fair play and team spirit.

8 Teaching Riders With a Disability

You do not necessarily need special training to be involved in teaching riders with disabilities. What you do need is to be knowledgeable and to have the right blend of confidence and understanding. All good teachers coach people, not sport. Working alongside disabled riders will be simply an extra challenge to your observation and adaptability.

Disabled people have been riding almost as long as their able-bodied counterparts. Over 2000 years ago the Greek horsemaster Xenophon used amputees, paraplegics and other wounded soldiers to carry messages on horseback to and from the Greek generals in battle. Ever since then horses have helped disabled people, not only as a means of transport, but also by alleviating their problems and broadening their horizons.

Riders in the UK first truly realized what they could achieve when Liz Hartell, a Danish rider, won a Silver medal for dressage at the Helsinki Olympic Games. This was despite the fact that Liz was partially paralysed in both legs from poliomyelitis and only able to walk a few steps at a time with the aid of crutches. However, this is not the place to chart the history of disabled riding. Suffice it to say that in the UK there are now over 26 000 riders and drivers registered with the Riding for the Disabled Association (RDA). The RDA is the sports organizing body.

What sort of disability?

This chapter is directed at the ordinary instructor dealing with a lesson for a disabled rider for the first time, rather than being a standard RDA text. For this purpose disability means a physical or mental weakness (or sometimes both) which may be either congenital (present from birth) or acquired due to accident or illness. It can be assumed that these problems are permanent, or at the very least, long term. The disability may be life threatening as in multiple sclerosis, permanent and unchanging such as an amputation or spina bifida, or as basic as arthritis, a bad back or epilepsy. Frequently the same condition can affect different people in different ways, for example cerebral palsy can affect half the body (hemiplegia), just the legs (diplegia) or the arms and legs (quadriplegia). Occasionally it can also include mental handicap. Whatever the problem, however large or small, the instructor has to work around it, not fight head-on with it. The instructor has to be aware of this added training difficulty, but not obsessed by it. Obsession with the problem tends to blind the instructor to the strong points and other weaknesses in the riding ability of the client.

A little thought about the terms used when referring to people with a disability may prevent embarrassment for the teacher and irritation for the rider. Avoid words such as 'handicap' or 'handicapped' and do not simply talk about 'the disabled'. Use terms that emphasize that these are people such as 'riders with a disability' or 'riders who are deaf'. It is useful to become familiar with some of the more common terms:

- impairment – a loss of use of a faculty or a part of the body which is either temporary or permanent.
- disability – a loss of ability due to the impairment.
- handicap – the physical barriers caused by the disability.
- amputee – a person who has lost one or more limbs or parts of limbs.
- hidden impairments – a wide group of conditions which in themselves do not directly impair movement, but may have a disabling effect on other body functions, for example, epilepsy or diabetes.
- *les autres* – a term of convenience used to describe all physical disabilities that do not fall into convenient categories, for example, polio.
- paraplegia – primarily the loss of use of the legs, usually because of injury to the spinal cord. The higher up the spine the injury, the greater the loss of body function.
- physical disability – an impairment directly affecting movement or the control of movement.
- sensory disability – affecting the senses.
- learning disability/difficulty – mental impairment is the most correct term but mental handicap is still commonly used. This

results in a person's intellectual capacity not developing as quickly or as fully as other people, leading to learning difficulties. Sometimes this arises from genetic abnormalities, for example, Downs Syndrome, or by infectious disease before or after birth.

Do not generalize; not all riders with the same type of impairment will have the same degree of disability. For example, cerebral palsy can vary in severity and in the range of mobility it allows.

It is strongly recommended that no disabled rider is taught without express permission from a doctor. The RDA insists on this for insurance purposes. A physiotherapist should be consulted about the rider's physical problems so that the instructor can be sure to use only exercises that will not harm the rider. It is often an advantage to have a physiotherapist present during the lesson to deal with specific problems as they arise.

Whatever the rider's handicap, the instructor must treat the rider in the same way as an able-bodied rider: first as a human-being, second as a rider and, lastly, and then only if it is relevant, the disability should be taken into consideration. Each rider and his/her individual disability must be viewed on his/her merits and treated just like any other client in terms of setting attainable goals. All preconceived ideas must be shelved when teaching a disabled rider for the first time and the instructor must teach what he/she sees, even more so than with the able-bodied rider. The riding instructor must endeavour to teach the disabled person to ride a horse to the best of his/her ability. Just as with able-bodied people, this ability varies from person to person, but this must not stop us aiming as high as is realistically possible.

Unfortunately humans, unlike disabilities, do not fit easily into categories, and when the two are combined each situation has to be evaluated on its own merits. It helps if the instructor has some knowledge of each problem and how it most commonly affects riders. With many of the physical disabilities it makes sense to ask the riders themselves what can and cannot be achieved. The instructor should also ascertain the goals and aspirations of each individual. Sometimes, however, verbal communication is not easy, but do remember that just because a rider does not speak it may not mean that he/she cannot speak or that the rider has hearing difficulties. Communication goes both ways! Remember that the vast majority of people with a physical disability do not have a learning difficulty.

When first talking to a rider the instructor must not be shy or embarrassed about discussing the problem or disability. The instructor will not be the first person, or the last, to ask and it is very important to be armed with as much information as possible before starting so that the lesson is as productive as possible (Fig. 8.1). The goals of mentally handicapped riders are usually different from those of the physically handicapped. Although different, they are just as important to the rider concerned, and the teacher or carer accompanying the rider should be brought into the discussion to ascertain these goals at an early stage.

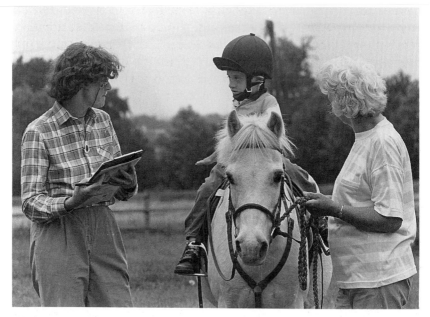

Fig. 8.1 Find out as much as you can about the rider and his/her disability. (*Courtesy:* Riding for the Disabled Association)

Whenever possible riders should be helped to fulfil their own ambitions, not our ambitions for them. The instructor should allow the riders to identify their own achievable goals, as only then can a training plan be drawn up, showing each progressive step with the short, medium and long term goals. This exercise helps the riders as they are in control of their own destiny.

When talking to riders in wheelchairs move yourself to their eye level when talking to them. This is polite and prevents you looking down on them. Remember that their wheelchair is often considered as an extension of themselves – do not use it as a prop for arms, legs or bags.

Mentally handicapped riders

The category 'mental handicap' is very wide and varied, so much so that it may mean very little to the riding instructor. Some riders, for example, cannot understand the concept of a circle, and yet would quite happily ride a rein-back or leg-yield. Their lack of spatial awareness has nothing to do with their riding ability, these are completely different concepts and must not be confused. Prior knowledge of the rider, from a parent, carer or teacher, is essential before starting.

When teaching mentally handicapped people the instructor must be very aware of the words that are used. You cannot say 'Hold on' one moment and 'Don't drop it' the next (Fig. 8.2). Be prepared to try several ways of saying the same thing until something clicks with the rider and then stick to that format. Be adaptable, but once a phrase registers, don't change it! Be aware that mentally handicapped people

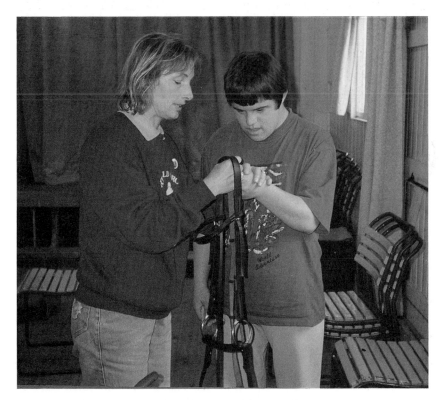

Fig. 8.2 When teaching mentally handicapped people be very aware of the words that you use. (*Courtesy:* Riding for the Disabled Association)

are often very literally minded and may not understand non-literal terms. Some may not be able to understand a negative command, hearing only the positive part, so that 'Don't lean forwards' is heard as 'Lean forwards'. They may also need more reinforcement of the things that they are learning; be prepared to go over things again and again, in the same order and the same words. Another thing to remember is not to allow a rider, especially a mentally handicapped rider, to get into incorrect habits, as they can seldom be corrected. Mentally handicapped riders with some understanding can almost be 'programmed' into riding well, even if they do not understand why they are doing what they are doing. This works particularly well during stable management sessions, as long as the instructor is consistent in what he/she says. Once riders learn, for example, how to rug up a horse the correct way, they cannot comprehend doing it the wrong way.

Frequently 'visualization techniques' are a beneficial way of teaching the mentally handicapped. Telling a rider to sit up straight may not register, but saying 'Come on, look smart, pretend you're a soldier' may get a completely different response. The pony may start to march faster too!

One of the instructor's main roles when dealing with mentally handicapped riders is to act as co-ordinator. In a ride of six, not only are there six horses and six riders, but there may also be six leaders and one or two side helpers per rider (Fig. 8.3). As safety is paramount, the instructor has the job of marshalling the ride. The instructor must be a good communicator and develop rapport so that he/she can control the ride and the helpers. Knowledge of the riders is of vital importance as problems such as an epileptic or asthma attack can occur very quickly.

Remember some people will never learn to ride, but that should not stop them sitting on a horse if they enjoy it or if their health improves. Bear in mind that those people who live in a Home benefit from simply socializing with a different group of people and from getting out into the 'big wide world'. This type of rider benefits from playing games on horseback, or even from just going for a ride in a field; it all gives the rider confidence, stimulation and freedom. Riding also helps balance and co-ordination; something as simple as doing up a coat button or a zip can be a very useful exercise, even if it is to help the physiotherapist and not the instructor. However, no exercise is useful if it puts the rider, pony, instructor or helper at any risk to their safety or dignity. Some riders would never understand that we are laughing with them, not at them.

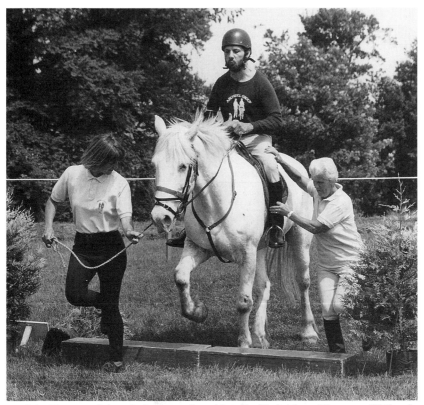

Fig. 8.3   Teamwork is a vital aspect of teaching disabled riders. (*Courtesy:* Riding for the Disabled Association)

Physically handicapped riders

Various problems can arise when trying to stimulate or motivate a rider. People who could ride before the accident that disabled them are often frustrated and this barrier must be broken down before progress can be made. People with a physical disability may resent what little they can do now because as an able-bodied person they could have done more. They may not try, saying 'What's the point?'. They may also resent everybody who is helping them, accusing them of being patronizing. This is seldom a fair accusation, but when one is 'at war with the world', every excuse for a negative response is seized upon.

Socializing is also very important for physically disabled people. They can discuss ideas and problems and learn to support each other; they then realize that they are not so different after all. For people who have suddenly become disabled, mixing with others can help them come to terms with their own problems. Children learn to make friends and cope, disabled adults with the same condition can teach young people far more about coping with their disability than an able-bodied person can.

There are no hard and fast rules about teaching disabled riders, and sometimes a trainer may appear slightly 'alternative' to get the desired results. Generally speaking, the phrase 'If it's safe and it works, it's right' has been of the most use to me in teaching the disabled to ride.

The choice of suitable horses and ponies

The primary teaching aid to learning to ride is the horse or pony. This may be stating the obvious, but very often not enough thought is given to the selection of horse, pony or donkey used for training riders with a disability.

Temperament
Old retired ponies are usually thought to be the best, but these older animals tend to be stiffer and more prone to unlevelness. Any animal that has a placid, unflappable personality can be considered. Avoid ponies that cough as the movement involved when the pony splutters disrupts the rider's balance and may unnerve the rider.

Movement
After temperament the animal's paces have to be considered; they should be as smooth and rhythmical as possible. Even more important than the paces, the pony should have transitions that disturb the rider's balance as little as possible. Small riders, or those with narrow hips or tight upper leg muscles, need a narrow mount as sitting on a wide pony may cause discomfort. Riders with balance problems do better on wider ponies as this gives them a broader base of support.

Weight
The weight of the animal must be considered and not confused with the weight-carrying capability. Remember that small riders can be placed on large ponies but large riders cannot be placed on small ponies. Small ponies have limited weight-carrying ability and short, choppy strides, which means that ponies under 13.2 hh may not get enough work unless they are driven as well. If horses are more than

16 hh, helpers may have difficulty assisting the riders once they are mounted and the sheer size can unnerve a rider who lacks confidence. Remember that whenever possible, whether the riders are beginners or more advanced, the horse should be better schooled than its rider. This means that horses and ponies should be regularly schooled or lunged by competent people who can train the horse, not for themselves, but for the riders.

Facilities

Mounting block

All disabled riders *must* mount from a mounting block of some description. This prevents strain on the horse's back and saves the saddle from being twisted or damaged. The block must be sited in a safe, enclosed area, preferably with a restraint on the right-hand side to prevent the horse moving sideways as the rider mounts. The block must be made so that the rider can mount from either side, as with some disabilities getting on and off from the 'wrong' side is imperative. Some riders have to lift their leg over the horse's neck and care should be taken to prevent their foot catching in the reins. The block height should be such that the top is level with the bottom of the skirt of the saddle and large enough to allow room for one or two assistants, as well as a wheelchair. A hand rail up to and around the top is necessary and the block should be accessed by a slope of no more than 32 degrees. Mounting and dismounting should be seen as part of the lesson, and all riders encouraged to achieve as much as they can without help, provided that they are safe.

Arena

After a suitable horse the next major requirement is for an enclosed area. This does not mean that riders always have to ride within four walls, but it is better, if possible, to start off inside a safe arena. A flat surface is desirable for the helpers, but as far as the riders are concerned, a slight unlevelness of the ground or a change of gradient can help their balance and start to teach them to adjust and control body movement.

Once established and confident in a safe area, the rider will benefit from riding in a field, progressing to riding through woodland and other terrain. This sense of freedom helps the rider's confidence and provides stimulation. So often the wheelchair-bound are never able to go through trees, over tree roots or through puddles. Just the act of ducking under branches, moving to look up at a squirrel or going up a slope assists balance and co-ordination. Instead of bending round cones in the school, why not weave in and out of some trees or bushes?

Tack

It is the duty of the instructor to use whatever means possible to help the riders achieve their aims. Our limitations should not limit those we teach. Adapt the horse's tack for each individual rider as and when it is necessary and relevant. However, do not get carried away; keep it simple.

Each horse or pony should wear a headcollar and lead rope, with a bridle minus the noseband on top. It is advisable for all animals to wear a breastplate with a leather handle stitched to it. The animal's usual saddle should be worn, with safety stirrups if the rider is not wearing the correct footwear. If there is a risk of pressure sores to the rider, a saddle saver should be added. Pressure sores may occur with riders suffering from circulatory and sensation problems or muscle wasting disease.

Some riders should not have stirrups as their feet coming into contact with a hard ungiving surface can cause their legs to go into spasm. If riders do suffer from involuntary muscle spasms it is of no use to tell them to keep their legs still. Equally, do not tell them to relax, for the opposite is likely to occur as the riders try too hard. To stop the riders having to worry about their lack of control of their legs, due to weakness or spasm, Velcro or elastic bands can be used to minimize the movement. This should only be done after consultation with the physiotherapist. It is essential that any modifications like this must be able to come apart or break easily, in case of an accident. Some wheelchair-bound riders glue a Velcro strip to the sole of their boot and to the stirrup tread so that they cannot lose the stirrup while riding. Many of these ideas will come from discussion with the riders who know their own problems better than anyone else.

Adaptations
Saddles can be adapted in a number of ways, for example, a side saddle with the fixed and leaping heads fixed to the off side, an ordinary saddle fitted with a bucket to accommodate the stump of the

rider's leg, a saddle with a leather strap on the pommel or a metal bar welded onto the tree to prevent the rider balancing on the horse's mouth.

General purpose saddles are more useful than dressage saddles as they are more adaptable. Whether they are synthetic or leather is a matter of personal choice, but synthetic saddles do have the advantage of being lighter. A Western saddle may be helpful for some riders. The deep seat gives a feeling of security and helps their balance; however, the high pommel and cantle may make mounting and dismounting difficult. Tightening a cinch when the rider is mounted is far more difficult than tightening a girth.

Reins are easily adapted, but before much money is spent on custom adaptations, remember that there is a large selection already available. Once a pair of reins has been adapted they may need to be used on a number of horses and it is a good idea to make the length adjustable at the bit end. As with able-bodied riders, reins should not be so long that the rider can catch a foot in them. If the rider has a problem telling left from right, why not buy coloured reins and have one red and one blue rein as a pair. Most riders will understand 'Pull the red rein'. Wearing one red and one blue glove accomplishes the same thing. Some riders with grip problems can cope with continental reins while others need ladder or loop reins. With mentally handicapped riders or those with uncontrollable arm movements, it is more considerate to the horse to attach the reins to the headcollar rather than the bit.

Thalidomide victims or other riders with short arms may need loops on their reins and a fixing onto the saddle or breastplate to improve the angle of the contact to the horse's mouth. If a driving terret is fixed onto a breastplate, the angle is far less harsh than if the fixing is clipped onto the D rings on the front of the saddle. Ladder reins are useful for riders who can only use one hand, but as with all these adaptations, both horse and rider have to get used to them. Whatever the design or material of the reins they must be the correct width for the rider as well as being comfortable, not slippery or rough. Any tack adaptations or aids must be relevant and continually reviewed. If the adaptation is no longer needed discard it.

Some riders wear callipers to help stabilize weak joints when walking. If their joints are at risk of damage without the callipers, they should not be removed for riding, but care must be taken to ensure that metal callipers cannot jam in the stirrups or damage the saddle. Callipers that run over the inside of the knee may need padding to prevent rubbing when the rider uses his/her legs. Full leg callipers may present a problem around the upper thigh and could necessitate an adapted saddle.

Artificial legs are designed for walking, not riding and they may not allow the rider to sit symmetrically. Some dedicated riders have a 'riding leg' which is specially designed so that they can sit in the correct position. If the rider has double short stumps it may be more effective to ride without the artificial limbs, and to fit the stumps into 'bucket sockets' hung from the stirrup bars. The decision to remove an artificial limb for riding must remain with the rider, as some may be sensitive about the amputation.

The other thing to bear in mind when discussing tack adaptations is the rider's feelings. Many riders do not like to be different and dislike the idea of having unusual equipment. Those who want to ride to the best of their ability will usually use whatever means available to facilitate their improvement. All this must be discussed with the riders and their helpers.

Teaching disabled riders

The teaching of disabled riders can be split into three sections:

(1) Hippotherapy
(2) Educational and remedial riding
(3) Riding for pleasure.

Hippotherapy
Hippotherapy is the treatment of a patient using the horse as the treatment modality. Conditions that involve disorders of balance and movement may be helped by using the movement of the horse to initiate a response from the patient, who may sit or lie on or across the horse in whichever position enhances the desired effect. While walking the natural free movement of the pelvis of both horse and human are the same. Therefore, sitting on a correctly moving base can, over a period of time, improve faulty balance and movement patterns in the patient, allowing him/her to function more effectively in other activities. Hippotherapy is best carried out with the patient on a blanket attached to the horse by a surcingle, as the warmth of the horse can be an important feature in relaxing tight muscles and stimulating circulation. While sitting on the horse at walk the rider's body performs up to one-thousand muscle contractions per minute in response to the

movement of the horse. Sometimes just the feel of a warm pony can make riders who live in their own worlds start communicating with the outside world.

Hippotherapy is not a recreation but a treatment and must be carried out under the direction of a physiotherapist.

Educational or remedial riding

Many disabled riders ride for the remedial effects and here the instructor and the physiotherapist need to work together. These riders do not need physiotherapy while on the horse as in hippotherapy, but remedial riding will improve their basic balance and co-ordination both at rest and while moving. It is a good idea to encourage these riders to ride outside as much as they ride in the arena . When they do ride in the arena it is useful for the physiotherapist to take part in the lesson. The physiotherapist can advise and help them with centring their position in the saddle, then with balancing their body above the centred seat. No matter what the disability, the centring of the seat followed by the trunk is the first priority.

The instructor's task here is firstly to monitor safety – he/she is in charge of the lesson. The instructor should also ensure that, as well as learning, the riders have fun, using whatever means are available. During the ride, basic stable management and theory can be introduced, even if it is as simple as 'What colour is your pony?'. Be careful with the wording of these questions; a Downs Syndrome child was asked 'What do you call a black and white horse?'. The answer was, of course, 'A cow'.

Lesson plan for remedial group ride

This is a very basic plan to be adapted and changed depending on abilities and aptitude of the riders. After every ten minutes of work there should be a short rest period.

(1)   Instructor and/or physiotherapist help the riders mount while an assistant alters and checks girths and stirrups, etc.
(2)   Start off with riders working on their own in walk with their leaders or helpers. Introduce transitions to halt to help with individual disabilities. The helpers should have been briefed already by the physiotherapist. During this time the instructor should be assessing, co-ordinating and maintaining the safety of the ride.

(3) After a short rest allow the physiotherapist to help with group exercises, preferably at walk.
(4) Improve the riders' steering by introducing school movements, bending in and out of cones at walk, gradually reducing the assistance from the helpers to a minimum, if any.
(5) Introduce practice trotting under the physiotherapist's advice and assistance.

During every rest period co-ordination exercises can be used with bean bags and rubber rings, or aspects of stable management could be taught. If the physiotherapist is not available, the instructor will take over all these activities backed up by an assistant acting as another pair of eyes.

The individual lesson
The best way of teaching the more advanced rider is to teach an ordinary lesson as though the rider was able-bodied:

(1) Warm up and assess problems.
(2) Discuss the lesson plan with the rider, highlighting the aims of the lesson, the rider's goals and problems.
(3) Use relevant exercises and movements to work towards the goals. Be aware that the rider may tire easily. If the physiotherapist is present enlist his/her help.
(4) Cool down and debrief constructively.

Riding for pleasure
Disabled people may ride purely for pleasure and recreation. These are the riders with whom the instructor can achieve the most in terms of riding improvement. They want to learn to ride for the sake of riding, and tend to be people who are physically or slightly mentally handicapped. This is where competition becomes beneficial as an objective means of demonstrating rider improvement. Although some riders do jump, it is more usual to aim towards riding dressage tests. Even if the competition is between a ride of six performing a very simple walk test, the achievement can be measured. There are now organized dressage events for the disabled at local, regional and national levels. Walk only lead rein tests are the most basic while the most complex are equivalent to BHS medium level dressage. Not everyone agrees with competition but it does give the riders something tangible to strive towards.

To give an example, a rider suffering from multiple sclerosis competed at a regional show and qualified for the national competition in both a class for first-time riders and in the freestyle to music. Afterwards she said, 'I was inspired, dressage is good for the poor old brain, you can't think of anything else while you are doing it, which I needed so badly. I am sure it has helped my ability to walk and my balance too'. Another rider said, 'I can be an athlete on my horse. I can't dance, the sticks get in the way, but I can do ballet with my horse'. She went on to win a Gold medal at the World Championships.

If riders enjoy competition it gives them an interest and a goal. We as able-bodied instructors must not restrict their ambitions as long as they are realistic and we do not concentrate on these riders to the detriment of the others.

Teaching the deaf

In this world of instant communication, being deaf has its own complex difficulties. For a start, it is an unseen problem, and people seem to be far more understanding of a disability that is obvious to everyone. Pick up a phone and you can speak to someone anywhere in the world. Go into any teenager's bedroom and music from a tape, radio or CD fills your ears. But, for many life is not like that. Born without the ability to hear, the deaf cannot easily acquire the art of speech and vocabulary, and so of course communication will always be a problem. More often than not, it is a problem for life.

Once the communication barriers are broken down there should be no reason for a deaf person not to learn to ride as well as any able-bodied rider. For many instructors the deaf are the most difficult (but not impossible) group to teach. You cannot instantly praise good work or correct errors and a lot of hand waving and exaggerated lip movements may be needed. The lesson style tends to be different and very often runs along the lines of:

- warm up
- stop and explain the lesson plan
- practise
- stop and comment
- practise
- improve
- debrief.

Having a hearing rider as lead file may prove helpful; it cuts out the need to explain to the deaf rider where to go. An able-bodied rider can also help by demonstrating school movements and errors and their correction. Learning sign language can be beneficial providing that the riders understand it, and not all adults do. British Sign Language and Makaton are the two types 'spoken', and most local authorities can advise on where to take a course. It is however rather difficult to talk in sign language while riding so conversation tends to be one way. Lip reading should not be overdone; just speak clearly and fairly slowly without exaggerating. Very often a good way of getting carers involved is to use them as interpreters and after a while you will develop your own way of communicating.

Teaching riders with sight problems

As with the deaf, riders with partial or total sight problems have their own special needs. How do you explain to a child how to ride a 20 m circle when he/she has never seen one and the only circle he/she has ever felt is a rubber ring? Try riding blindfold (in safe surroundings) and get the feel of what it is like to control an animal when you are lacking a basic sense and relying totally on your instructor. Human markers calling out the letters in the school as the rider approaches them can help, as can drawing the shape of a movement on the rider's hand. Many blind riders talk a great deal, as without sound their world goes away. Touch, feel and normality are vital to these riders and they are very sensitive and can pick up anxiety in your voice or touch. Blind riders depend on your confidence.

To keep the whole thing in perspective, try to explain a colour to someone without saying 'It is the same colour as...', 'It looks like...'. Try closing your eyes and touching all the parts of a horse and then joining them together to make a coherent whole – you will not be able to but it gives an insight of the problems involved.

Riding for the Disabled Guidelines for teaching groups with visually impaired riders

Before riding starts
Find out from the school, centre or rider the type of visual impairment, whether from birth or from later brain damage or illness. Ask if there are any other difficulties, for example, lack of spacial awareness,

impairment of hearing, problems of orientation or learning difficulties which affect ability to understand and carry out instructions.

It is important to establish the amount of vision and the particular problems of each rider, for example, short, long, blurred or tunnel vision and if the rider is affected by conditions of light or shade. If the rider has had sight in the past, he/she will remember colours, for example. Otherwise he/she will have nothing to recall to make mental pictures.

In the riding school

Introduce yourself by name with a firm hand on the rider's shoulder rather than a handshake. Introduce the riders to the ponies, allow them to examine in detail the one that they are to ride, particularly its height, and allow them to feel its breath and soft muzzle.

Describe the saddlery and any other equipment used, including the mounting block and invite them to feel everything you have described, particularly the length of the reins. Discuss the area where the riding is to take place and, if appropriate, ask them if they want to walk the area. Having established their capabilities, make sure that the riders are treated tactfully and as normally as possible and that their abilities are respected. Always ask them how best you can help them.

Always address the riders by name and identify yourself during the lesson. Remember that once they are familiar with the riding area and trust the instructor and helpers, they will make the same progress as seeing riders. It is necessary to make the lessons interesting and varied; it is easy to become bored when you cannot see your surroundings.

For partially sighted riders, use large signs and letters, above ground level. Poles and markers should be white at the top and bottom with contrasting colours in between. White reins could be useful.

During the lesson

- Give riders time to get their bearings in the riding area. Never push them and always be ready to lead them.
- Use precise language and a clear voice. Directions must be explicit, for example, 'Turn right at E, you are approaching it, turn right now and ride to me here in the centre'. Use the words right and left only as directional instructions, not in their other meanings.
- Guide riders through actions with your hands showing them how to use their reins for steering and how high to rise to the trot.

- Give time for instructions to be understood, and prepare riders in advance for corners, turns or stopping.
- Before jumping, walk the course with the riders and let them feel the height of the jumps. Only experienced instructors should teach jumping.
- Avoid sharp turns and small circles.
- Riding instructions should come only from the instructor. Helpers must not confuse riders. If necessary helpers can repeat exact verbal commands for changes of direction, for example. Timing is most important.
- A helper wearing a bright coloured hat, scarf or jacket walking in front of the pony may help. Ask the riders how best you can help them to use the sight that they have.
- Elastic bands can be put on the reins at intervals positioned for different riding requirements.

Starting at the walk, teach riders to count the paces, then teach them how to halt, using the correct aids and position. They will learn to count the strides round the arena. Each week teach something new and try to make use of music. Make sure there are bleepers for the markers and use a bell or a whistle to get the riders' attention. Always familiarize the ponies with these sounds before the riders are mounted.

Motivation and competition

Motivation is the key to training. Motivation is where the trainer, mentor or guru can excel; indeed it is sometimes the trainer's main job and is summed up in the following way. Motivation:

- gives insight;
- gives opportunities for skill development;
- forms and develops a pattern of behaviour.

In order to accomplish this the coach will:

- develop awareness by the gathering of appropriate high quality knowledge;
- encourage the pupil to take responsibility for the training (self motivation);

● effectively question to discover the extent of the pupil's knowledge, understanding and improvement.

The role of the coach is to guide pupils in the right direction and help them realize their full potential. At the same time the coach must remain honest about that potential and not encourage the riders to believe that they are something they are not. Thus the coach has to encourage his/her pupils to 'GROW':

G   goals
R   realistic aims
O   opportunities to achieve
W   weaknesses (and strengths) that are likely to affect short, medium and long term aims.

The riders who achieve most are those who can motivate themselves. If the trainer has to do all the work, he/she will become very frustrated and have less time to give to other people. Riders who lack motivation often benefit from a revision of the goals which may result in them concentrating on a less taxing area. To give an idea of the commitment and effort needed for high level competition, here is the general plan for three years' training for international riders.

The British team returned from Denmark in 1991 with fairly mediocre results after the second World Championships for Disabled Dressage Riders. A completely new training approach was taken in preparation for the 1994 World Championships to be held in Gloucestershire. Instead of the riders coming together for the occasional competition and demonstration, monthly training sessions were held. These started two-and-a-half years prior to the Championships. The sessions were for any likely team member, so that as many riders as possible could be assessed. Any riders not likely to achieve team status were given advice on where to go for extra help and their progress was monitored. The more serious contenders were trained at these monthly sessions by some of the country's leading trainers for the able-bodied.

The sessions were designed to help the riders and their usual trainers and gave the riders a chance to develop into a tightly knit group. Some very strong friendships developed and from an early stage each rider formed a good team of supporters. The riders exchanged health tips and ideas for sponsorship so that a good team spirit emerged. This sort of interchange is vitally important to success at whatever level of sport is played. Two intensive five-day courses were held each year and these training camps covered aspects such as test riding, what judges look for, care of the horse at competitions, sports psychology and mental rehearsal techniques. As part of the competition involves riding borrowed horses, part of the training was riding as many different horses as possible.

Prior to the Championships, a five-day Selection Trial was held to make the final team selection of eleven riders. The Selection Trials were held over this long period to observe how the riders coped with the prolonged pressure. On the first day all the riders who wanted to be considered for the 'own horse' team rode an international dressage test, judged by British Horse Society List 1 or 2 judges who had not been involved in the training of the riders. Three days were spent riding strange horses before the trials for those wishing to compete in the 'borrowed horse' category. In competition, riders have seven to ten days to become accustomed to their borrowed horses. The team selections were then made bearing in mind ambassadorial skills, ability to perform under pressure and the ability to be part of a team, as well as riding ability.

Training was then intensified to include test riding, coping under pressure and advanced lessons under the tutelage of two Fellows of the British Horse Society, the Chairman of the able-bodied dressage selectors, other List 1 judges and a sports psychologist.

As well as attending these organized sessions the riders continued their training at home, with some riding four or five times a week on borrowed horses. Bearing in mind that many of the riders were not just disabled but also in pain, this was no mean feat. The team included riders with muscular dystrophy, cerebral palsy, spinal injury and open pressure sores. One rider endured a spell in hospital during the training period and another could ride for no more than ten minutes at a time. It is obvious that the five individual Gold Medals, the Team Gold and the Team Silver were won as the result of a long hard fight, commitment and courage.

Rewards and achievements

Teaching physically handicapped riders has its own challenges and frustrations, which are quite different to those of teaching mentally handicapped riders. The two skills are different and some instructors find it easier to do one, some the other, but there is no reason why an instructor cannot excel at both. Remember that physically disabled riders tend to become frustrated when their bodies will not obey them. Success tends to come from overcoming or working round a problem, to enable horse and rider to perform to the best of their ability. The body might be weak but this does not mean that the mind is weak as well; the wheels on a wheelchair help the person move, they do not help them think! Riders often improve as understanding improves, despite their inability to achieve physically.

The abilities of mentally handicapped people tend to be different and so they must be taught differently. Much of the time they would not comprehend the concepts involved in learning to ride – they just do it! These riders need to be stimulated and to have fun. They cannot be taught to ride a circle if they have no understanding of shapes, and for some it may take a long time to grasp the idea of rising trot – but at their level of ability, this is a great achievement. Those who are also physically handicapped may need to spend time doing exercises on horseback, but these should always be fun and can incorporate the use of rubber rings, bean bags and anything else that is safe and stimulating. Where possible these exercises should be carried out at walk as balance and co-ordination are improved by using the movement of the horse. Ponies, riders and helpers will all get cold standing around in winter.

Teaching and working with the disabled riders revolves around developing a trusting relationship, regardless of the ability of the rider and the expertise of the trainer. The trainer has to know when to push and ask for more, and that only comes from working with and observing the rider for a long period of time. The instructor must be aware immediately of secondary problems that can trigger a rider into being difficult, weaker or more tired than usual. If this happens the instructor must know when to back off and to accept less than would otherwise be expected. Much can be achieved at the walk, and it is better to achieve three good ten minute sessions a week, than one worsening session of half-an-hour.

Riders must have confidence that even if they do not feel that a particular aim can be achieved, if their coach says that they can do it, then they will try their best. The rider should be encouraged to 'have a go', as long as it is remembered that there is always tomorrow, and a rider must never be rushed or forced into a frightening experience. The risk factors must be controlled and acceptable, just as in any 'thrill', and must be balanced with safety, which is paramount. If riders are encouraged and allowed to achieve then the 'sky is the limit' as the medals from the 1994 World Championships prove. At whatever level, and whether improvements are made or not, if the activity is safe and the riders enjoy themselves, the instructor has achieved a great deal.

9 Teaching the Novice Adult

First of all we need to establish why an adult wishes to 'learn' to ride. Do they really want to learn or do they simply wish to acquire a modest degree of skill? One could ask if these two aims are indeed the same; however, they are probably not. 'Learners' are usually people who want to understand thoroughly the skill that they have set out to master, either because they have some ambitious target or because that is their nature. On the other hand some skill can be learned without an indepth understanding of the subject.

Let us consider factors that may inhibit the learning process of a novice adult. To all beginners horses seem to be very large and if a person has no previous experience or familiarity with horses their sheer bulk can be frightening. It is therefore worthwhile spending some time familiarizing the client with the horse and helping the client to understand the horse's instincts and natural behaviour patterns. The reasons why certain bits of equipment and tack are used and the reasoning behind the chosen method of instruction are also valuable additions to the introductory lesson. It is often advantageous for adults who are considering learning to ride to watch another beginner lesson to help them begin to understand the 'language' and the format of this sort of lesson.

Fear can stem from many sources, for example, the fear of the pain caused by falling off or simply from severe discomfort experienced when riding. These fears need to be discovered and allayed as far as possible. The fear of a fall can be helped by using sufficient explanation and direction throughout every stage of the learning process and by adhering to sound, safe teaching practice. It is more difficult for the teacher to be aware that the rider is experiencing discomfort and it is useful to look at sources of discomfort and pain.

Clothing is a frequent cause of the problem and the riding instructor can help advise on suitable clothing for the beginner rider. A BSI current standard hat is a 'must' whether owned by the client or by the riding school. The hat must fit securely; if it is loose it will be distracting and hazardous. Shirts or jumpers should fit to allow unrestricted, comfortable movement. Trousers are a key item; if too tight around the crutch they are extremely uncomfortable for male and female riders. Equally underwear should give adequate support where necessary. If trouser legs are too loose they will ride up and pinch or rub. Shoes should have a well defined heel unless suitable safety stirrups are used. A boot, short or long, is more suitable as it provides ankle support. Provided that the client finds them comfortable and they are not too thick, gloves can prevent blisters.

Remember that beginner riders will be using different muscles which are not fit, and it is sometimes difficult for the regular rider to remember how quickly these unfit muscles tire and become sore. The teacher must be aware of this and plan the lesson accordingly.

Fear of failure or ridicule is very significant. As a teacher, remember the difficulties you encountered when last mastering a new skill, always try to set achievable goals and never be sarcastic or short-tempered. The teacher must be particularly careful when teaching groups that the competitive tendency of the participants is kept under control so that no one is made to feel inferior.

Teaching a novice adult in a riding school is in many ways easier than teaching someone who has gone out and bought a horse that may not be suitable. The riding school, however, must ensure that the horse selected for the client is a suitable size and shape and familiar with the level of work demanded. The saddle must also fit the client with leathers and irons of a suitable size.

Most clients benefit most from individual lessons until they are competent to walk, trot and canter in an enclosed area. Lunge lessons are ideal as the horse is controlled by the teacher and a close rapport between rider and teacher can be developed. It can also be very comforting for the rider to realize that you, the teacher, are in control of the horse. You can demonstrate this to pupils by allowing them to watch you warming up the horse before they mount. Attention must be paid to the size of the circle, preferably keeping the horse out on a 20 m circle. Initial lessons should last no more than 30 minutes and always leave the rider wanting more.

Teaching a person to mount is sometimes difficult and the use of a mounting block will avoid the horse being abused. A mounting block may not be necessary if the horse is small and the rider athletic. Throughout these early lessons demonstration is a useful aid to learning as is having a valid reason for teaching something a certain way. Thus the novice adult should not just be told to hold the reins in a certain way or to adopt a particular position in the saddle; the teacher should also explain why these things are done that way. At each stage check that the rider has fully understood what has been said and encourage the rider to tell you how he/she is feeling as the lesson progresses. It is essential that the rider feels confident in his/her ability to start and stop the horse with relative ease, so these simple but vital aids need plenty of practice. The horse's tack should include either a neck strap or breastplate, particularly when the rider is attempting to master rising trot.

It is recommended that the first steps of trot are sitting to help the riders become aware of how the horse is moving underneath them. The riders should be encouraged to hold the neck strap and to find a comfortable place in the saddle to sit. Remember throughout that the riders must not be given too much to think about at once; they need to be able to focus on one target at a time. The first lesson may not need to go beyond this point. Each individual should be allowed to progress at his/her own rate and the instructor must be most vigilant to ensure that this progression is logical and fulfilling . A record should be kept so that the instructor knows exactly what point has been reached and on what horse. Ideally the same instructor will take the rider through all these early lessons to encourage bonding between pupil and teacher (Fig. 9.1).

When the rider is proficient in walk and rising and sitting trot, he/she can be allowed to ride off the lunge and to build up steering skills. Any difficulties encountered should be worked through to build confidence and to increase the rider's repertoire of skills and reactions. At this stage it is probably a good idea to begin to introduce the 'what if' scenarios: what if the horse does not go forward from the leg?; what if the horse does not respond to a turning aid?; what if the horse fails to stop when asked?; what if the horse shies or bucks? If the teacher suggests ideas to the rider as to how he/she should try to react, it may prove useful in an emergency.

How to introduce canter to the novice rider is always a tricky problem. The method chosen depends largely on the qualities of the individual horses used for this exercise. Just as extremely well balanced, smooth and obedient horses can give the rider much confidence on the lunge, the calm obedient horse will give confidence when cantering round the school. The vital fact is that the experience of cantering gives both confidence and enthusiasm. Once the rider feels happy cantering, riding in a group can be an enjoyable experi-

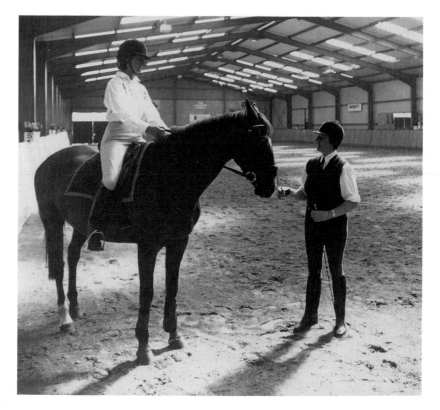

Fig. 9.1 Bonding between pupil and teacher is essential for confident progress.

ence, especially if the group ride together on a regular basis and the social aspects of the sport begin to be enjoyed. Proficiency in group riding can now be developed, so care must be taken to explain how horses behave in groups. Agree the rules of group riding and ensure that everyone adheres to these rules at all times.

When each rider in the group can ride his/her horse as an individual, for example, they can walk when everybody else is trotting, or they can turn away from the group, then they are probably ready to progress to riding outside. This can be in the field or out on hacks; if the hack includes road work a short talk on traffic procedures and courtesy to other road users is useful and can prevent an accident caused by ignorance or thoughtlessness. The riders should also be warned of the procedures to be followed in the event of an accident occurring during the hack.

At a trekking centre where beginner riders are simply taken for a slow ride in walk, not all these early learning steps may be necessary.

However, it is still recommended that some assessment of the fundamentals of riding takes place to ensure that the horses provided are suitable for the people who are to ride them. To this end a competent supervisor should watch the riders mounting, check their stirrups and girths and then observe the ride in the pace at which the ride is to be conducted. Ideally this assessment should take place in an enclosed area. If there is any doubt whatsoever as to the compatibility of horse and rider, the combination should not leave the premises.

Let us return to our serious learner who may wish to expand his/her competence. This may include riding up and down hills or even jumping; whatever is chosen, each stage should be clearly explained and taught in easily assimilated chunks.

The golden rules for teaching novice adults are:

- Riders should progress at the speed at which they feel confident.
- Safety and good practice must be top of the teacher's list of priorities.
- The teacher must be enthusiastic.
- Each pupil must feel important (Fig. 9.2).
- For many adult learners the social aspect of riding is important; if

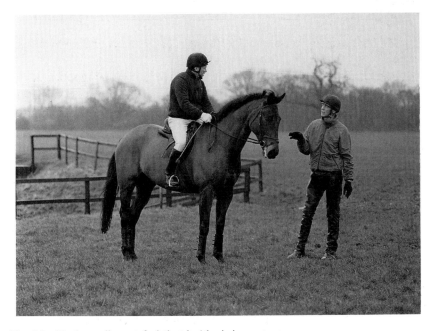

Fig. 9.2 Each pupil must feel that he/she is important.

they want to discuss their children, home, clothes or politics, the teacher should show lively and responsive interest.

For example when we go to the hairdresser, we are all aware that it is important that the assistant who washes our hair chats and shows an interest in us. Those of us who deal with the general public in our day-to-day teaching must develop ourselves to improve our communication skills. We must never allow ourselves to be surly or disinterested.

10 Coaching for Competition

Whether training individuals or teams for competition, the first thing that must be established is the goal. If the goal is achieved we have 'won' even if the rider did not take first place.

Coaches and competitors have to be matched to perfection to enable continuing success through confidence and security in the training system (Fig. 10.1). Horsemen are athletes, and can suffer from injuries and consequent setbacks.

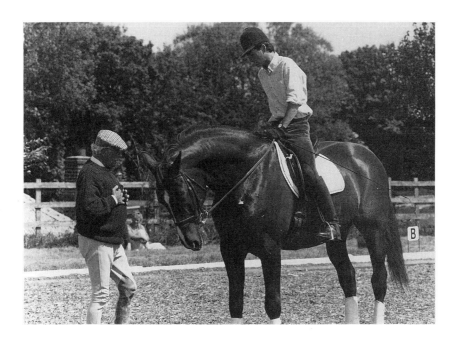

Fig. 10.1 Coaches and competitors have to be matched for success.

Building winning partnerships

Consider first the personality of the competitors. Do they need motivating by an external force, usually the coach, or are they highly motivated? If they need motivating the coach must ask him-/herself, 'Am I a motivator?'. Perhaps we should analyse what is meant by this. A definition could be 'to stimulate action'. The competition coach needs to be able to do this; can you? The answer is 'of course you can!', any competent teacher does this all the time. For example, if a horse will not settle in the dressage test and needs to be lunged beforehand, can you persuade your pupil that this is necessary if improvement is to be achieved? To accomplish this you may initially have to offer to help with the lungeing; when success is beginning to show then your rider will probably take over on his/her own. Once you have suggested a course of action some riders will immediately act upon it, but it can be difficult if you have a rider who constantly finds reasons for not trying out new techniques. It may take all your tact, diplomacy and confidence to ensure that your riders are prepared to take action and to follow this action throughout.

Motivation is also about providing incentive. Normally the incentive for competition riders is provided by the possibility of achieving their ultimate goals, whatever they may be. The goal may be as small as reducing the dressage score from 40 penalties down to 38; alternatively it may be as ambitious as to qualify for Badminton. The incentive may be provided by the coach but great care must be taken that the coach is not using the rider for his/her own ends. An example of this may be that the coach would like to have a horse compete at a major championship and therefore encourages the rider to aim for a qualifier for which he/she is not equipped, either technically or mentally. This can be a great disincentive if the competition turns out to be a failure. Equally if the pupil is aiming too high, it is the job of the coach to negotiate a more suitable goal.

It is important to try to avoid negative experiences such as competition failure. In so doing the coach must not give negative advice but must try to word the changing of the goal in such a way that the pupil thinks it is his/her own idea. In many ways we are luckier than some sports coaches because we have a lot of ammunition in the cupboard: the horse and his technical, physical and mental state; the venue and its likelihood to bring out the best in horse and rider; the opposition – who are they and what are the chances of beating them? If we are training jumping riders we can also consider the course and its complexity, while with dressage the complexity of the test and the suitability of the riding surface are all factors to put to the rider.

At this stage we must already be alert to the psychological effects of asking too much of the horse. Although the horse may perform well on the day, the signs of stress may not appear until the next competition and the horse's performance begins to deteriorate. There are several ways to avoid this situation.

Adequate training

Try to ensure that both horse and rider are trained so that the competition comes well within their current scope, for example when competing at novice dressage level, the horse should be working towards elementary at home. Consistently schooling over large fences is not recommended, but from time to time jumping 3 in higher than is required in the ring is a real boost in keeping both horse and rider confident that they can easily cope on a competition day.

There are exceptions to these guidelines, for example one does not normally school over Olympic size fences prior to the competition. On these special occasions horses of Olympic calibre often 'pull out all the stops' and perform up to and beyond their normal parameters. The same applies to events such as Badminton. Lucinda Green, when asked what made a Badminton horse, replied 'One that comes through the flags at the finish'. Sometimes one sees a horse that is not enjoying the competition; his ears are back and he has to be ridden hard by his rider. This horse may complete the competition, he may even jump a clear round, but the experience will have left its mark. Both trainer and rider must be aware of this and take careful action if the horse is to continue to compete successfully in the future.

Strategic planning

Having seen that our horse and/or rider have been stressed unreasonably the trainer must consider carefully what to do next. If possible the combination can drop down a grade in competition to give them an 'easy' run. This is easy to achieve if the horse is still eligible to compete at the lower grade, for example, we may decide to run an Advanced-graded event horse in an Advanced Intermediate class in order to monitor the horse's reaction. This can be essential if it is nearing the end of the season and there is a likelihood that the horse will upgrade and then have to start the new season in the new grade without any experience of more advanced competition. Although there are special competitions to help overcome this, they may not be strategically placed in the competition calendar of your horse and rider, nor may they be geographically well located to suit your competition needs.

Schooling at the competition venue
If it is not possible to drop down a grade then try to arrange a schooling session at a competition venue, to rebuild confidence, evaluate performance and to decide on the future course of action.

Assessing the cause of stress
It goes without saying that the trainer and rider must analyse all possible causes of stress. Is the problem due to a lack of:

- talent?
- technique?
- training?

Is the horse fit for the job?

- Has he a good temperament?
- Does he travel well?
- Has he been off colour recently?
- Are there any indications of injury or pain?

Both trainer and rider must agree on one rule – if the horse or rider are not 'fit to compete' for any reason, they must not do so. Even if they have already travelled a long way to a competition, commonsense and horse-sense must prevail. One often sees riders at a competition apparently with no-one to turn to for help and advice. An example of this occurred at a three day Horse Trial several years ago; a young competitor came into the ten minute box, his horse was clearly stressed and both the veterinary surgeon and the Ground Jury felt that he should not continue. When approached and advised that 'there is always another day' he was aggressive and unwilling to accept the decision, however, authority prevailed. As he led his horse back to the stable area it had a severe nose bleed and would certainly have collapsed had the competitor continued the competition. While this was a salutary lesson, how sad for him that he did not have a competent coach to help him through his disappointment. In international competition there is a Code of Conduct to which all riders, owners, grooms and trainers must adhere (see Appendix 2).

A further example of causing unwitting distress is described in the following scenario. The rider was a very keen amateur with some talent, especially across country. He was highly motivated and liked to discuss each aspect of the overall training in great detail and to have an indepth evaluation of each competition performance. He was not easily defeated and might carry on at times when it could be wiser to give in.

His horse was very talented and graded Intermediate, but a tricky customer, often inclined to nap on exercise, although usually quite co-operative at competitions. The horse was rather tense and difficult in the dressage, inclined to become strong and exuberant in the show jumping and bold and strong across country.

The trainer was very experienced and had trained many horses and riders at International level. He enjoyed 'discovering' and fostering new talent. On this particular occasion the horse performed an average dressage test and went clear show jumping. The cross country started well but then the horse dropped the bit and was reluctant for the rest of the course, eventually being pulled up. The rider thought that the horse was being disobedient and was very despondent; however, the trainer thought that there must be a reason for this uncharacteristic behaviour. Rider and trainer evaluated the 'what can be the matter list?' mentioned earlier and could draw no firm conclusions. It was thus decided to blood test the horse when he got home. The rider and trainer travelled home together from the competition during which time it was important for the future that the trainer continued to identify the 'good' that had been achieved and to have the confidence that a remedy could be found.

The horse was found to be dehydrated and had been extremely distressed. This affected the horse psychologically such that it never performed to the same level again. No one was to blame and a great deal was learned by all concerned, indeed much progress has been made since that time with respect to the problem of dehydration. However, the rider needed a great deal of help to get over the feeling of being a failure; he felt he should have known and pulled up earlier but his rationale during that competition was quite understandable.

The trainer and coach have a vital role to play in times of stress and disappointment. We are there to help at all times, not just the good.

The equine coach is not always as accustomed to travelling to the competitions as an athletics coach may be. However, all coaches should try to see their pupils compete at some time in order to gauge the reactions of both horse and rider to the competition environment.

If the pupil does not ask the coach to participate in the competition experience until there is a major competition on the horizon, it may not be possible to make the changes in competition technique that are necessary for success. Equally, the competitor must not be so dependent on the coach that he/she cannot perform without the coach being present.

One of the roles of the competition trainer is to discipline the riders to carry out procedures as agreed. They must also be able to take appropriate action if the rider does not follow the agreed procedures. The key word here is 'agree'. The coach must ensure that they agree the goals, the technique, the route, the strides, the speed and other factors. The coach must not dictate what the rider is to do. It is likely that young competitors will need more leading towards the agreed procedures than experienced competitors, who may simply want to clarify their own decisions. Between these two extremes lie a large number of riders whom the coach will be able to assist in developing a clear plan of the procedures to follow in various situations.

Several years ago there was a qualifying competition for the Junior European Show Jumping team. The track was built the night before and it was nearly dark before it was ready to walk. There were about 50 competitors in the class and as our rider was first to go the coach decided it would be beneficial to walk the course in detail that night and then to walk it again quickly the next morning to refresh the mind. While the course was being built there was a party in full swing, but our keen coach and rider left the party and walked the course, which was large and complex, the most difficult our rider and her horse had tackled so far (Fig. 10.2). The coach realized this but was keen that there should be no doubt in the rider's mind as to her ability to cope. Great care was taken with the line between the fences, the strides to be taken through the related distances and the amount of impulsion needed through the doubles and combinations. The discussion on the technique to be followed was mostly coach-led due to the inexperience of the rider, but once agreement was reached they retired for the night. In the morning they walked the course again with the rider telling the coach how she was going to tackle the course, and any doubts or hesitation were talked through so that the rider was completely sure what she was going to do. The result was a clear round, the rider was able to ride the course exactly as planned and everybody was delighted.

However, what should the coach do when the agreed strategy does not take place? This happens quite often and each time the coach and rider must both ask 'why'? No competitor wants to make a mistake

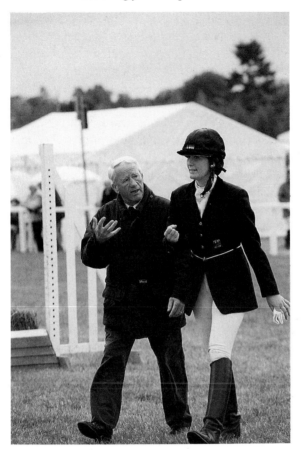

Fig. 10.2   Walking the course. (*Courtesy:* Elizabeth Furth)

deliberately; competitors are usually very disappointed with their own performance when success, or an agreed goal, is not achieved. The coach must stand back and give the situation some time before starting to talk through the problem. I have had personal experience of being 'attacked' on leaving the ring, having had a fence down, and this did not enable me to perform better. Indeed one owner was so well-known for his tirades that people made a point of stopping to listen!

Consider the following scenario: the coach agrees with the rider that her goal is to go clear and within the time at a three day event (Fig. 10.3). The horse is both fit enough and experienced enough to be able to achieve this. Coach and rider agree where the rider has to be on the course at certain times to allow her to monitor her progress. However,

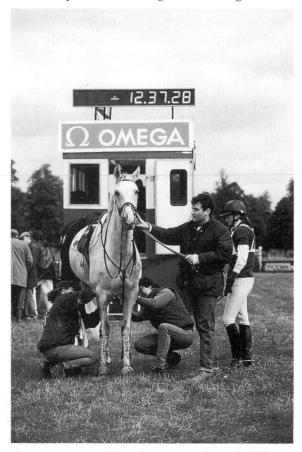

Fig. 10.3 Agreeing the goal with the rider at the start of the steeplechase. (*Courtesy:* Elizabeth Furth)

it is obvious by the time that the horse and rider are half way round the course that the goal is not going to be reached; the rider is having to set up the horse carefully for the jumps, and this is very time-consuming. When the rider finishes she knows that she has gone over the time and is very distressed because she feels that she has not only let the coach down, but also the owners, the groom and all her supporters. At this point it is part of the coach's role to reassure the rider and to look at the successful aspects of the round; that the horse jumped well and clear and that all the agreed routes were taken. After the horse has been cared for the coach can sit down with the rider and quietly discuss what went wrong. On this occasion the horse had become unexpectedly strong and the rider had felt that she could not allow the horse to gallop on in case she could not get him back and set the horse up sufficiently for the obstacles. The way forward is for the coach and rider to discuss tactics to reduce the possibility of this happening in future competitions.

If the rider repeatedly makes the same mistakes, such as misreading his/her stopwatch, the rider must be encouraged to wear a watch more often and to become accustomed to making accurate readings at all times. If the rider always shortens a horse in the show jumping so that it takes more strides than the course builder intends, further training must take place to eradicate this tendency and to develop the rider's confidence so that he/she allows the horse to stay on the correct stride.

The most difficult situation for the coach is when the rider becomes very tense and nervous and makes mistakes as a result, especially in the dressage phase. For these riders, the preparation outside the arena during the warming up is vital (Fig. 10.4). The reactions of the horse and rider as a combination must be studied. If the horse has a nervous

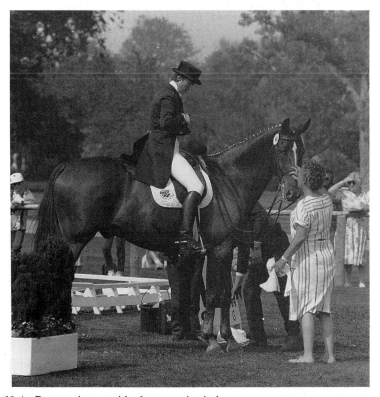

Fig. 10.4 Preparation outside the arena is vital.

temperament or has a history of 'blowing up' in the arena, then working for a maximum sparkling performance when warming up may be detrimental. How much chance to take in psyching up horse and rider has to be carefully estimated and agreed with the rider. Only by having previously accompanied the rider to competitions can a suitable strategy be reached. There are times when the coach may have made a mistake or an incorrect evaluation of the situation, and the coach must be prepared to admit this, but not to the point that the rider loses confidence in the coach's advice.

I do not believe it is ever productive to be sarcastic, disgusted, abusive or dismissive when debriefing riders after competition. Certainly agree what must be done to try to solve a problem or to improve performance but always be *positive* (Fig. 10.5).

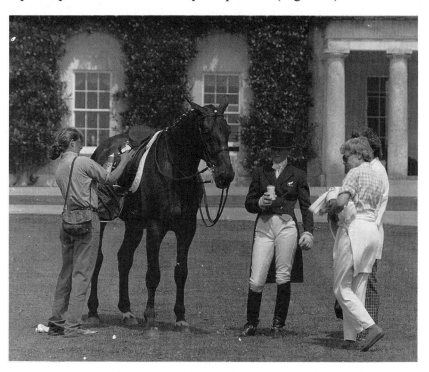

Fig. 10.5   The debrief must be positive.

For some riders mental rehearsal can be helpful (Fig. 10.6), indeed most riders do this to some extent already, for example when walking a course. This technique can be especially useful for riders that find the dressage phase nerve-racking; the rider not only memorizes the

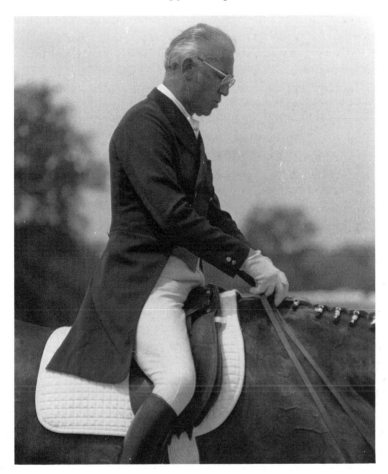

Fig. 10.6 Mental rehearsal by the rider.

test but also plans how to ride the test movement by movement as follows:

- Enter the arena area. The horse settles best in canter, on the right rein and there is about two minutes warm up time before the judge rings the bell; this will allow two circuits of the arena. If the horse is settled move the horse on for a few strides and then back to working canter. If he is a little tense stay in working canter and reassure the horse with voice or a pat.
- The horse will anticipate the halt, therefore the entry must be at a purposeful canter and do not ask for the transition until the marker.

- The move off must be purposeful, setting up the bend once we move off; this will help the medium trot.
- The medium trot will be rising to encourage the horse not to hollow and hold back.
- The downward transition must be positive; with the shoulder-in already in mind ride through the corner with purpose to avoid loss of impulsion.
- Flow into the 10 m circle, maintaining impulsion.
- Ride one straight stride before the half pass as the horse is inclined to lead with his quarters; keep him flowing all the way to the centre line.

This can be continued through the whole of the test, leaving as little as possible to chance. If there are any areas that the coach suspects may cause particular difficulty, it is useful to go through the 'what if' scenario, for example, 'what if the horse refuses to rein back?'. Is the rider going to insist on achieving the movement, abandon it or compromise? What the rider and coach agree will depend on that individual horse and rider.

Mental rehearsal is of particular importance in the ten minute box at a three day event. Ideally, the rider and coach should have time alone together (Fig. 10.7), unless it is a team competition. Coaches have to consider the needs of each individual rider. They will have been monitoring the performance of other competitors so that they can advise their riders on their return to the box. There are four possible scenarios as follows.

(1) The easy situation is when the course is riding well and no adjustment to the riding plan needs to be made, the rider will simply go through the course and rehearse the riding plan.

(2) It is more difficult when the previous competitors have fared badly but the mistakes are spread around the course; then the coach must keep the rider confident in the agreed strategy. The coach must assure the rider that the horse is fit and capable and that the course is not riding badly, it is simply that other riders have made mistakes and that the rider is well prepared and will not experience any trouble.

(3) The third situation occurs when tactics have to be changed because an agreed route is jumping badly. The coach must thoroughly brief the competitor on the change of route and ask the competitor to talk it back. Above all the competitor must set

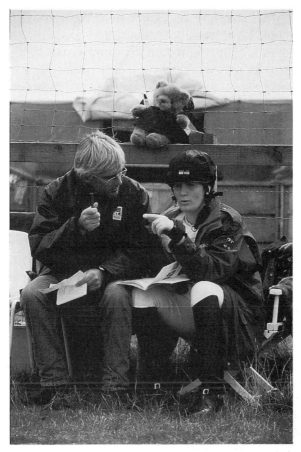

Fig. 10.7 Mental rehearsal in the ten minute box with the coach. (*Courtesy:* Elizabeth Furth)

out sure and confident of what he/she is going to do and how he/she is going to ride the course.

(4) The most distressing situation is when another horse has been injured and there is a delay in the box. The coach must minimize the tragedy and keep the rider's mind occupied with positive thoughts. If the delay is prolonged, remind the rider of other successful rounds that have taken place. The rider may want to talk to other riders but do not encourage conversation with unsuccessful competitors. Every horse and rider is different and it can be confusing to listen to conflicting stories and advice. However, the coach should see and listen to as much information as possible and then select the relevant information to give to the rider.

It can be tempting to ignore or ridicule observations from others but I personally once learned a sharp lesson; I was jumping at a county show on my good Grade A mare and was eliminated at the water; this was a problem occasionally and I was pretty cross. As I left the collecting ring an old horseman said, 'Ah, t'was the sun glinting on the water did put her off'. I thought he was a silly old fool until I discovered a year later that the mare had a cataract. A very humbling experience!

A coach and a competitor need to 'gel' to be a successful team but partnerships are not achieved over night and instant success is unlikely. Some competitors change their coach every time their performance is unsuccessful – this is not recommended as it does not allow time for consolidation of the partnership and just because one competitor is successful with one coach does not mean that this success can be repeated in every case. I would hate to think that the equestrian world is like football teams which seem to change coaches and managers with alarming regularity.

Coaches working together

Due to the nature of our sport coaches often work together from an early stage. To be successful this requires an open-minded, sharing attitude. At one level there may be the Pony Club rider who has a regular instructor but when he/she goes to a rally he/she has a different teacher. There is nothing worse for a teacher than when a pupil in this situation says, 'Oh, but my instructor says that's wrong and I should do it this way . . .'. There are two points that need to be addressed here:

● The child should have been advised already that he/she may be asked to do things differently, that he/she must co-operate with the new instructor and that any differences will be discussed and future action agreed.
● The instructor at the rally has to handle the situation with tact, never criticise other teachers, listen to the child and then explain why he/she has offered conflicting advice.

If the same child gets into a Pony Club team he/she may then have a different team trainer. The wise trainer finds out who the child's regular instructor is and does not try to change anything but simply builds on what is good and makes suggestions to improve the weaker areas. The open-minded regular instructor will recognize when useful advice has been given and gratefully accepts this.

A further 'sharing' situation arises when a rider has one coach for the dressage and another for the show jumping. Ideally both coaches should share ideas so that there is no confusion for the rider. If possible it is useful for each coach to watch the other work and if conflict seems likely they should discuss the problem and try to negotiate some sort of compromise.

The other likely scene is where a competitor is selected for a team and the team coach is expected to prepare the competitor at the competition. In this case the daily trainer can talk to the chef d'equipe or the chief selector and discuss whether he/she should be involved. In most cases the chef d'equipe's main concern is that the team should perform successfully and if, by including the rider's trainer, the chances of success are improved he/she is likely to encourage the daily trainer's participation.

It is essential that the coach is fully aware of the rules of the particular sport.

What makes a successful competition coach?

The following are all essential qualities and all coaches should work on them in order to enhance their effectiveness:

- enthusiasm
- empathy
- skill at the sport
- skill as a teacher
- skill as a motivator
- knowledge of the sport and its rules
- patience.

Psychological preparation for competition

The successful competitor usually views competing as a way of life with different rules and standards and different demands and expectations. As most people become competitors voluntarily most of the pressures are self-inflicted and expected. The fact that you choose to compete separates you from the non-competitor. However, everybody in this elite will be an individual and different, just as the demands of competition will be specific and different. Regardless of the type of competition, certain criteria are the same. These are:

- a desired level of fitness to attain;
- a higher level of skill to reach;
- a required commitment of time and energy;
- an optimum training method and programme;
- an attitude to training, competition, other individuals and problems that arise which will all affect success.

Both coach and competitor have to predict stress and anxiety. Primary stress is related to the task in hand and the competitor has to learn to cope with it. Secondary stress is usually outside the competition and is brought in by external concerns such as family, money, etc. These worries should be left behind and not allowed to interfere with success. This is often difficult for the individual and he/she may need help and encouragement from the coach.

The effect of anxiety on competition performance

In order to help the competitor the coach must be able to recognize the rider's sources of anxiety. These may include:

- risk of injury to horse or rider;
- threat to self esteem, for example losing or falling off;
- pressure to perform beyond one's perceived capabilities, for example competing in an intermediate event when not ready to;
- lack of preparation or training, for example the horse or rider are not fit enough;
- living up to the expectations of other people such as the trainer, parents, friends, team mates;
- fear of failure, such as losing a competition when in the lead.

These fears will result in anxiety which may be expressed as:

- negative expectations or thoughts;
- worry;
- lack of concentration;

- disrupted attention;
- decreased self confidence;
- increased heart rate and sweating;
- tense and heavy muscles;
- butterflies in the stomach;
- irritability;
- withdrawal from crowds;
- decreased motivation.

Unless the coach recognizes these signs, which will vary in each individual, and acts upon them, the competitor's performance is likely to suffer because anxiety will:

- cause tension in the rider. This will be transmitted to the horse resulting in a stiff and tense horse;
- reduce a rider's attention and irrelevant thoughts may crowd his/her mind. This leads to bad judgement and errors will follow;
- cause the rider to doubt his/her own ability and reduce self confidence, resulting in poor performance.

Some of the solutions available to the coach include:

- awareness of rider's anxiety level when competing;
- relaxation techniques;
- positive thinking – stop negative thoughts;
- concentration techniques;
- positive self talk;
- goal setting;
- imagery;
- psyching-up techniques.

The method chosen will depend on both the coach and the competitor as well as the reason for the anxiety and the sport in which they are involved.

11 Preparation for Teaching Examinations

No matter what sphere of the horse industry you are involved in, there is no substitute for experience. Teaching is no exception. It is unwise to have total responsibility for lessons prior to qualification, and some teaching under supervision is essential. The supervision can be direct with your trainer watching you teach or could be through guidance with your lesson plans and help with any problems that arise. Success at examination will depend on the candidate having:

- studied the syllabus thoroughly;
- acquired the necessary knowledge;
- participated in as many teaching situations as possible;
- ensured that his/her riding skill is sufficient to be able to demonstrate adequately;
- studied different teaching techniques;
- studied how people learn;
- practised lesson planning;
- implemented lesson plans;
- developed powers of observation;
- practised examination technique.

The syllabus

The Preliminary Teaching Test is the first step up the instructional ladder and is offered to members of the BHS; full details can be obtained from the Training and Education Office (see Appendix 1 for teaching plans). The syllabus is a short leaflet and requires some expansion, for example it states 'Candidates must show that they have the required qualities, and can apply the basic principles of teaching, e.g. manner, voice, control, etc., and that they have the ability to improve their pupils' horsemanship and horsemastership with a progressive plan'.

Manner

The candidates must have the ability to communicate as we have discussed. They must also present the required demeanour and appearance. The teacher, especially in a commercial riding establishment, must command respect by being tidily and suitably dressed for each individual situation. He/she should exude enthusiasm for the customers by smiling and making them feel welcome – remember the customer is always right. Equally, the voice should convey warmth, enthusiasm and sincerity.

Voice

Effective use of the voice is an essential technique that should be developed during teaching practice. Some teachers have abused and over-used their voices to such an extent that they have suffered permanent damage and had to stop teaching. Arguably riding teachers place more demands on their voices than anyone other than a drill sergeant; projecting one's voice for sustained periods requires considerable training and practice, especially when teaching outside and battling with the elements or external factors such as traffic noise or machinery. Teaching in the summer or indoors where the surface becomes dry and dusty poses a potential hazard that can be very harmful to the voice. Even if you are a confident teacher with naturally good voice production, your voice has to be looked after if it is to stay the distance. If the teacher lacks confidence or has a strong dialect or accent then the chances of the pupil mishearing or misunderstanding are increased. Ideally try to get some help from a drama teacher.

Normally during the exam two people are teaching at the same time and this must be practised to enable you to gauge how much extra effort you are going to have to put into producing your voice effectively. The riding teacher should avoid straining his/her voice so that if you have a cough, cold, sore throat or croaky voice you should try to cut your teaching load by as much as possible or alternatively use amplification. Part of the riding teacher's training should encompass the use of microphones; such equipment has been developed to allow direct communication between rider and teacher for use indoors and outdoors. If you are teaching for several hours at a stretch, you should have frequent drinks of water; however, the inclemency of our weather means that we tend to fall prey to excessive intake of coffee, tea and drinking chocolate!

Control

Who and what are we controlling? Ideally the teacher is in control of the whole situation – horses, riders and, where applicable, onlookers. Safety is of paramount importance; riding is a risk sport and it is the teacher's responsibility to minimize that risk while still enabling the pupils to progress and enjoy themselves. By planning ahead and setting realistic goals we can go a long way towards minimizing risk. Developing our powers of observation will help us spot potentially hazardous situations and to take action to avoid them. For there to be control there must be discipline; this is especially important with children who are less aware of the dangers of 'horseplay' around their ponies.

The preliminary instructor has to be capable not only of teaching in a controlled environment but also of escorting hacks in the countryside with due regard to safety and the necessary organizational requirements. According to current BHS requirements instructors also need to be trained and certificated in first aid. The would-be instructor will have already obtained the Riding and Road Safety Test as part of the Stage II examination which is a prerequisite for the Preliminary Teaching Test. Figure 11.1 shows the structure of the BHS qualification and examination system.

Knowledge

The candidate should have a clear understanding of the organization of a commercial riding establishment including:

- dealing with enquiries;
- processing bookings;
- making initial riding assessments;
- allocating horses to riders;
- organizing clients into rides;
- dealing with difficult customers;
- dealing with financial aspects such as receiving payment from clients;
- the benefits of class and private lessons;
- implementing the safety policy;
- care of customers after the lesson;
- incentive schemes for clients and teachers.

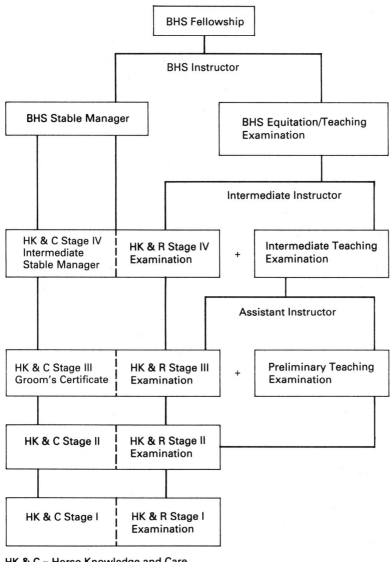

Fig. 11.1 Structure of the BHS qualification and examination system.

The preliminary teachers are not expected to be able to run a business on their own but must be capable of being left in charge for short periods. Their knowledge and understanding should be sufficient to reassure the examiner that they would be able to do this.

Teaching

The candidate will be expected to give a class lesson to three or four pupils working towards Stage III level equitation. To prepare for this the candidate must have had considerable experience with classes of between three and six pupils, lasting between 30 and 60 minutes. The pre-planning of lessons is vital and knowing how to adapt these plans to meet the needs of each client is an essential part of being a successful teacher.

In the examinations handbook published by the BHS there is a list of subjects which the candidate may be expected to teach in this section of the exam. I would recommend that a lesson plan is designed for each of these briefs. Remember, the plan does not replace the need to teach, it is the mechanism which enables effective teaching to take place. The teacher will still have to observe the ride and make suitable corrections to both horses and their riders. If the whole plan cannot be carried out in the limited time available in the exam, this is not a disaster; the essential point is that the candidates must always teach what is in front of them. There are 37 suggested lesson briefs and every candidate should have taught every one of these at least once. Remember to apply the basic principles of teaching outlined in this book throughout all the teaching situations.

Another key area of the syllabus is teaching the beginner rider (child and/or adult) either on the lunge or the leading rein. These aspects have been discussed earlier in this book but it is pertinent to stress the need for the teacher to build up the rider's confidence and to develop the correct techniques whilst having fun, safely. Further guidelines and lesson subjects can be found in the BHS examination handbook. The candidate should have had experience of teaching both children and adults in order to ensure competence and a positive result in the preliminary teaching test.

Once again it is recommended that all the subjects are planned and practised. I would like to stress that the lesson plan for the lunge lesson, in particular, should remain very flexible. Until the pupil has been assessed, suitable exercises cannot be selected. It is a good idea to keep a record of the exercises that you have found to be most suitable for various problems that the rider may be experiencing, for example if the rider tends to round the shoulders it is useful for the rider to rotate the arms and shoulders backwards. If the candidate uses exercises that are not relevant to the pupil, in other words the candidate does not teach what is in front of him/her, he/she will almost certainly fail the examination.

Equitation theory

It is also stated in the syllabus that the candidate should have a sound knowledge of basic equitation. This can be interpreted to mean a thorough understanding of the training of horses from breaking to novice dressage. The candidate would be expected to teach the classical position whilst evaluating, understanding and making allowance for the physical limitations of each individual rider. A basic knowledge of the structure and function of human anatomy helps to clarify this complex subject. The effects of the saddle and the conformation of the horse are also relevant to the teaching and understanding of the rider's position and should be studied by the candidate. The candidate should also understand the training of the horse over show jumps and cross country fences. Candidates should be able to discuss the production of horses and riders for novice competitions involving fences up to 3 ft 3 in (1 m) in height. This includes an ability to explain what is meant by the balanced jumping seat. Sound knowledge of the jumping distances used in training and in competition is essential.

This knowledge requirement is an expansion of that outlined in the syllabus. The intention is to enable the candidate to be able to discuss with confidence the basics of equitation and to give an insight into future progression.

Giving a lecture

The preliminary teacher must be capable of giving lectures on theory both in the classroom and in a practical stable management situation. Although the lecture given in the exam will only last for five minutes the candidate should practise delivering lectures of 15 to 30 minute duration. The purpose of this part of the exam is to give the examiner a chance to see how the candidate would handle a class in this situation. Again planning is the key to success; if the candidate has planned well he/she will have enough confidence in the subject to deliver a good lecture. The candidate must position him-/herself so that the audience can see clearly; this is very important when a demonstration is being used. The lecturer must capture the attention of the audience and this is best done by eye contact – look at the audience so that each pupil feels included and important. Again a list of lecture subjects can be found in the examination handbook.

Developing teaching techniques

Developing teaching techniques demands a lively and enquiring mind and candidates must make the most of any opportunities that present themselves, including studying their own instructors, teachers and lecturers and noting their good points as well as the weaker areas in their techniques. Go to lecture demonstrations and assess how well the presenters communicate with the audience and their pupils. Study videos and read books on communication skills and other supporting skills. Through this book you will have explored the basic ways in which people learn and how they acquire skills; these principles should be applied to your everyday teaching. Studying the skills of teaching is a lifetime's work and there is always something new to be learned.

Developing powers of observation

Our powers of observation can be developed outside the riding school; if you drive a car it is essential to be observant if you are to avoid an accident. Test others on how observant they are; it is surprising the things that are not noticed or are taken for granted. The eye becomes more educated with experience and knowledge and the observant eye of the stockman is the basis of good horse care. The dressage judge has to develop and educate his/her eye to a fine degree; if you have the opportunity sit in with a judge and assess if you can see the same, or even more, than the judge does.

Examination technique

A candidate's examination technique is developed through:

- studying the examination handbook;
- practising the lessons to fit within the allocated time;

- attending training days aimed towards the Preliminary Teaching Test, particularly those taken by examiners;
- participating in mock exam days;
- acting as a 'guinea pig' for Preliminary Teaching Test exams.

Ideally at least six months should elapse between taking the Stage II exam and the Preliminary Teaching Test; it is even better if candidates attain their Stage III before the preliminary teaching test. For more mature and experienced horsemen these recommendations do not necessarily apply.

Guidelines for the Intermediate Teaching Test

The Intermediate Teaching Test expands and moves on from the Preliminary Teaching Test; the basic teaching criteria remain the same and the candidate's structure of study can include the same foundation skills. The BHS publish guidelines for the Intermediate Teaching Test, which should be read in conjunction with this book. Normally access to this examination is via progression from the Assistant Instructors Certificate; however, more mature instructors of 25 years or more can apply for direct entry, backed up by a suitable curriculum vitae. The overall aim of this examination is for candidates to demonstrate that they are capable of training a horse and rider for elementary dressage and to coach a rider for Novice horse trials according to the requirements of the BHS. The Intermediate instructor should be capable of training students up to the standards of the BHSAI examination.

During the examination the candidate will be expected to:

- teach a lunge lesson;
- teach a class lesson;
- teach a dressage lesson;
- teach a jumping lesson;
- give a lecture.

The lunge lesson

This session will last 20 to 30 minutes. You must be able to lunge a horse very competently in order to be able to make your rider the top priority. In addition the horse must be a good lunge horse that suits the rider, as a horse going poorly will directly affect the ability of the rider to sit well enough. The examiner will observe your handling of the equipment as well as the quality of the lesson and will be looking for:

- correct handling of equipment;
- rein contact;
- whip handling;
- adjustment of the side reins;
- size of circle;
- awareness of the horse and distractions.

The overall aim of the lesson is to improve the rider's position, depth and feel. You must have a clear progressive plan that is sufficiently adaptable to respond to the individual needs of each pupil. Introduce yourself to your pupil and remember that the pupil, too, may be nervous. Find out the pupil's previous experience and whether he/she is accustomed to lunge lessons and ask the name of the horse. Check the horse's tack, establish its age, sex and conformation and then lunge it for a short time to assess:

- degree of obedience;
- level of training;
- the rein on which it lunges most easily;
- balance;
- impulsion;
- rhythm.

If the going is suitable give the horse a canter. It should be lunged without side reins initially and then the side reins can be fitted once the horse has loosened up a little. The side reins should be fitted so that when the horse comes into contact with them, the nose is just in front of the vertical. Often horses are a little lively without the rider but once mounted settle down quite quickly. This warm up and assessment should take no more than five minutes. Try to involve your pupil while the initial warm up is taking place.

The horse can then be halted, the side reins unclipped, the pupil mounted and the stirrups altered. The lunge lesson then begins in walk on the horse's best rein. The rider must start the lesson with both reins and stirrups so that his/her riding can be assessed, both in terms of the rider's position and the effect on the horse. Once the rider has settled in walk and feels confident on the lunge, you can proceed to rising trot. The horse and rider should be seen in walk and trot on both reins before you get too deeply involved in correcting the rider's position. The rider can now be asked to go into sitting trot. Look for the rider's ability to:

- stay supple;
- maintain an even rein contact;
- maintain position.

This work in sitting trot will help you identify the main area to be worked on. Try to identify the root of the problem and choose relevant exercises that will help that particular problem. Any exercises used must relate directly to the rider in front of you and his/her specific problems. Do not lunge on too small a circle except for a specific purpose and try to keep the horse's impulsion without losing the rhythm so that the rider has the best opportunity to improve. Keep the lesson safe but ensure that there is progression.

It is usual to take away both reins and stirrups in this lesson but do not take away both the reins and the stirrups at the same time. Depending on your assessment of the rider you may choose to take away the reins and allow the rider to become accustomed to the feel of riding without reins before taking away the stirrups as well.

During these exercises the rein should be changed every five minutes or so. The rein can be changed by leading the horse across the circle or the rider can turn him using a large pirouette.

If the rider does not have any major positional faults to work on then you can develop some more advanced work such as:

- transitions;
- introductory lateral work;
- increasing and decreasing the pace;
- increasing and decreasing the size of the circle.

However, in the exam situation you have only 20 to 25 minutes for the whole lesson and the time tends to pass very quickly. Once you have been told to bring the lesson to a close, give the pupil back the reins and stirrups so that you can note any improvement made. You can then halt the horse and ask if the pupil has any questions before giving the pupil some points to work on for the future. Finally the side reins should be unclipped, the pupil dismounted and the stirrups run up.

The class lesson

The class lesson requires an ability to teach, organize and keep enthusiastic a group of students working at Stage III level. Many of the aspects already outlined can be incorporated here; however, as time is short, it is not always possible to be student-centred in the approach so the lessons are likely to be tutor-led. The lesson should be both interesting and stimulating, and some account needs to be taken of your 'slot' in the day, for example, if you are first to go the exercises are likely to be more basic whereas later on the class will be warmed up and able to be taken on further. Usually about four riders are provided as guinea pigs. The lesson will either cover dressage work or grid work and will last about 25 minutes. It is essential therefore that the candidate is well practised in setting up a grid with help, in order to progress the ride without too much time being spent moving fences. The teacher must be clear and confident regarding the distances to be used with a mixed group of horses and should use fences up to around 3 ft (0.9 m) in height.

It is essential to follow all the guidelines given in the section of this book dealing with the class lesson, paying particular attention to the need to look after all riders as equally as possible. If you are the second person to teach it is important that your lesson is progressive and if you feel that there are any grey areas left by the previous candidate you should clarify these points in order to progress the lesson satisfactorily. Lesson plans need to be clearly thought out and it is a good idea to go to the exam with some to hand; examples can be found in Appendix 1. Drill exercises are permissible in this section but must contain good corrections, not just 'directing the traffic'. This means that you must be well practised at this sort of instructing in order to be able to concentrate on the pupil. Bear in mind that you will not know the horses or the pupils so it is vital that they understand the proposed exercise.

The positioning of the teacher is most important. You need to be placed so that:

- the pupils can hear you;
- the examiner can hear you;

- you can observe the ride from the best angle for the particular exercise being carried out.

The dressage lesson
The dressage lesson lasts for 35 minutes and includes some discussion time. It is vital that the candidate teaches what is in front of him/her. The aim is to progress towards Elementary level dressage, but if this is not possible do not panic – providing that progress has been made the examiner will be satisfied, so long as the required knowledge is demonstrated in discussion.

Once again it is important to introduce yourself to your guinea pig and to try to establish some rapport, even under difficult exam conditions. Find out about the pupil's previous experience and how well he/she knows the horse. Tell the pupil that you would like to use the first five minutes to assess both horse and rider, and ask the pupil to show the horse in walk, trot and canter on both reins. If capable of more advanced movements the pupil could show these briefly as well. If there are other horses in the school make your pupil aware of them and remind him/her of correct school procedure. Do not try to teach during this assessment period but do communicate – ask how the pupil feels the horse is going and how this compares with how he/she would expect the horse to go under normal circumstances. During this time you should assess the horse and rider and their way of going, including:

- the paces;
- balance;
- suppleness;
- temperament;
- standard of training and riding.

This will enable you to decide what to teach.

Once you have assessed horse and rider you should ride the horse for five minutes to establish if what you feel backs up what you see. Do not try to school the horse; the purpose is simply to feel how responsive the horse is to further clarify his training needs and to assess where the difficulties lie.

Once you have assessed both horse and rider you can agree with the pupil what to work on. Do not choose something the horse or rider find very difficult; it is not wise to try to tackle a problem that is going to need several months to put right. It is better to improve another area while drawing attention to the main problem and explaining how, with more time, this could be tackled. Remember, first and foremost, the horse must accept the bit and then work on the bit before he can perform any dressage movement correctly.

This lesson is primarily to improve the horse, but if the rider has a positional fault which is seriously inhibiting progress it must, of course, be addressed, but do not give a rider lesson at the expense of the horse. As you have used 10 minutes for assessment, you will have about 20 minutes left to teach the lesson. At all times ensure that you keep the pupil's interest and treat him/her as an equal – never talk down to the pupil. Conversely try not to be intimidated; remember that you are in charge and you must have the confidence and belief that you are going to help this horse and rider. It is essential that the examiner can hear you, so position your pupil so that this is possible. Although you may be sharing the school with another candidate, address most of your comments when your pupil is at your end of the school and take care not to disrupt your opposite number's lesson – just communicate as needed.

As with any individual lesson there must be a suitable beginning, middle and end and the needs of the pupil must be considered throughout. It is helpful if, prior to the day of the exam, you have practised teaching a lesson in the time available so that you are confident that you are not either going to run out of time or, alternatively, run out of things to do. Be careful when the examiner tells you that you have another five minutes left that you do not panic and try to cram everything into those last few minutes. Continue with your plan; if you have not got as far as you had hoped then admit it and apologize, explaining what you had intended to cover. Once you have been asked to finish the lesson, finish with something the combination do well. Try to debrief using the positive, for example asking them 'Which part of the work just done pleased you the most?' is better than 'Any questions? No, well thank you, goodbye'. Remember to give the rider some work for the future. The examiner will then talk to you, giving you the opportunity to discuss any difficulties you encountered.

To be properly prepared for this section you need to have had considerable experience teaching competitors on their own horses as well as matching combinations that have not worked together before. However careful a centre may be there are times when the guinea pigs are less than willing, and part of being a teacher is trying to overcome this uncomfortable situation. Be prepared to teach in all weather conditions and appreciate the effects of the weather on your pupil, the horses and the examiner.

Jump teaching

The jumping lesson lasts about 35 minutes and the basic strategy of this lesson is similar to the dressage lesson, inasmuch as the horse and rider must first be assessed on the flat. The examiner will have introduced him-/herself to the guinea pig and established the level of the horse and rider and what problems the rider would like help with. The examiner will then brief the candidate regarding the time available, the equipment and help available, and will introduce the rider to the candidate.

Throughout the exam the examiner will ask him-/herself several questions:

(1)   Does the candidate:

- attempt to set up some rapport with the rider?
- give the rider time to ask questions from time to time?
- give the rider short rest periods?
- praise the rider?

(2)   Has the lesson got a structure with a progressive plan and a clear goal?

(3)   Is the rider clear throughout what the candidate wants him/her to do?

Although there can be no ideal plan as every horse and rider requires different techniques, there are some guidelines. Initially assess both horse and rider on the flat. Ideally the rider should have given the horse adequate time to settle and work in before the lesson. The assessment should check the horse's:

- balance;
- acceptance of the aids;
- suppleness;
- temperament;
- paces, especially the canter.

Remember that the canter is the most vital pace for the jumper and normally a whole lesson in trot would not be acceptable. The introduction and flat work warm up should last no longer than 10 minutes.

The candidate should not jump in and start to teach immediately but stand back and observe horse and rider. Judicious questioning should enable the candidate to assess the combination's strengths and weaknesses.

Discuss with the rider his/her experience and aims and if there are any specific problems. Progress to an assessment of the horse and rider over fences. The height and complexity of the fences used during this assessment will depend on the experience of both horse and rider. However, the lesson must always be safe, and the examiner will stop the lesson temporarily if necessary to maintain safety. Normally the candidate would see the horse jump a small fence from trot and canter on both reins – a simple fence such as a cross pole or small upright would be suitable. A placing pole would not be used at this stage as this would not give an accurate assessment of the natural ability of horse and rider. It is essential for the candidate to make a verbal assessment at this stage and to explain the progression plan to be used in the lesson to the rider.

If the combination is harmonious and in balance the rider's technique should not be radically altered. However, if the rider is hampering the horse's progress then judicious alterations can be made. The candidate may ride and jump the horse if he/she wishes to.

The aim of the lesson is for the candidate to enable the rider to show some improvement. To this end the candidate can use any exercise, providing that the rider understands the exercise. For example, in the jumping lesson the distances should be suitable or the exercise designed to improve a specific aspect of the horse's or rider's technique. As you progress through the lesson check that the rider is happy and confident to use each exercise. Remember safety is the top priority. Unless the rider is exceptionally nervous or the horse is very green, try to progress towards fences of Novice Horse Trials or Newcomers standard, whichever is applicable to the combination in front of you. It is not essential to jump a course, the main objective is to improve the technique of horse and rider and to help them solve any current problems. It can be difficult to work on the horse if the rider is inexperienced or nervous. However, the examiner will allow for this in his/her assessment of the candidate's performance. The examiner will also be open-minded; the way the candidate chooses to teach may not reflect the examiner's own methods, but this should not influence the outcome of the assessment. Finish on a positive note and give the pupil clear pointers for future work.

If the horse is very excitable and you feel that jumping out of canter would be detrimental, discuss this with the examiner so that all parties have agreed the goal of this particular lesson. If flat work is necessary to make improvement, take some time after the initial assessment to work on the pupil and the horse but then return to the jumping to check that progress has been made. The fences must be handled with confidence and dexterity to enable progress to be made as smoothly as possible (Fig. 11.2). Whenever you are busy moving fences, give your pupil some work to do, do not leave him/her wandering about aimlessly. Take into account the going, especially if the ground is hard or slippery, when planning your lesson.

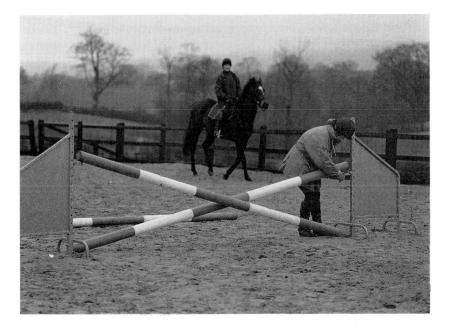

Fig. 11.2 The fences must be handled with confidence and dexterity.

Questioning

At the end of the lesson the examiner will question the candidate to find out:

- why the candidate used certain exercises;
- what homework the rider has been given;
- where the candidate would go from here, i.e. what the next lesson would consist of.

The examiner is likely to probe any answers given. For example, if the candidate replies 'I would work him down grids', the examiner will ask 'What sort of grid?' and expect to be told pace, distances and height of the fences.

If the candidate volunteers information about specific competitions, e.g. Foxhunter, then the candidate must be able to back this up with knowledge of the height and type of fence involved. Rules tend to change every year, so both candidate and examiner must be up-to-date.

Candidates must know the distances they have set up and the likely effect on the horse. They should not be afraid to admit, during the course of the lesson, that they have made a distance a little too short or too long, and to alter it accordingly. The distances in Table 11.1 can be used as a guideline to suit most horses. These distances are not competition distances, they are for schooling exercises.

Table 11.1 Jumping distances suitable for most horses.

Placing pole to a fence (trot and canter)			
bounce	8 ft	2.6 yd	2.4 m
one canter stride	19 ft 6 in	6.5 yd	5.8 m
Between fences (trot or canter)			
bounce	12 ft	4 yd	3.7 m
one stride	21 ft	7 yd	6.4 m
two strides	33 ft	11 yd	10.1 m
three strides	45 ft	15 yd	13.7 m
four strides	57 ft	19 yd	17.4 m
Pole on the landing side after a fence	12 ft	4 yd	3.7 m
Canter poles	9 ft	3 yd	2.7 m
One non-jumping stride between poles	12 ft	4 yd	3.7 m

Common schooling exercises the candidate might use include the A-frame, descending parallel or parallel cross poles. However, the candidate must always avoid building fences with a false groundline or kicking a pole under the fence to create a false groundline. Fences should never be jumped from the wrong side, in other words with the filler away from the horse.

The ideal lesson will lay a firm foundation for progression towards improvement. This will be achieved by the lesson having:

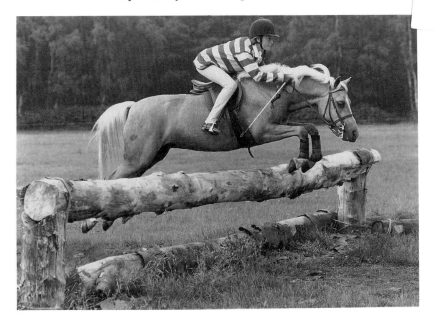

Fig. 11.3   A good horse and rider are only so in mutual trust.

- a clear structure;
- a progressive plan;
- a target;

and containing:

- safe practice;
- good teaching technique;
- a sound understanding of the training of both horse and rider.

The lesson should be stimulating and satisfying to all parties involved: the horse, rider, teacher and examiner. Remember 'a good horse and rider are only so in mutual trust'.

Throughout the exam, in any of the teaching areas, if you are concerned about either the horse or the rider, for example if the horse looks unlevel, talk to the examiner and discuss how to proceed. In preparation it is highly recommended that you sit in with dressage judges up to Elementary level or Intermediate Horse Trials level. It is also extremely useful to assist a course builder at a jumping show or to help a jumping trainer during teaching. These experiences help develop your confidence and further your knowledge.

The three remaining areas covered by the examination are giving a lecture, business management and training the horse. The lecture should be suitable for those working in a yard or preparing for their Stage III Horse Care exam. These lectures are short, lasting only five minutes, but as with the Preliminary Teaching Test the candidate should be confident to lecture for 30 to 40 minutes in order to show a sound lecturing technique and confident handling of the audience. A list of suggested lecture subjects can be found in the examination handbook.

Candidates can prepare for the section on training the horse only by practising their ability to discuss the subject, it is no good being very practical and experienced if candidates cannot express their opinions in discussion. The candidate must be well read and have a thorough understanding of training techniques. In discussion it is important to be sure of your own viewpoint without being dogmatic. Do not be afraid to disagree with another candidate providing that you can put forward a reasoned argument for your difference of opinion.

The Intermediate teacher should also be a good manager of people and have a thorough understanding of business administration. The examination of this section takes place through discussion.

The British Horse Society Instructor Examination

This exam consists of three parts: stable management, riding and teaching. The equitation and teaching must be taken and passed on the same occasion.

The dressage lesson
The dressage lesson lasts about 40 minutes and should involve movements up to Medium standard with a single flying change being introduced in 1996. The format is very similar to that of the Intermediate exam except that the level is higher and the teacher is expected to be able to cope with problem horses and riders and capable of overcoming nerves. The candidate should have a progressive plan for each lesson to enable a constructive lesson to take place. Just as in the Intermediate exam there should be an initial discussion with the pupil followed by an assessment of horse and rider; this assessment will be by observation of the combination and by riding the horse. This will

allow the candidate to choose a suitable aspect to work on and improve.

As before, sitting in with dressage judges at the required level is invaluable. In addition attending clinics, seminars and conferences will build up the teacher's repertoire and constant study and revision is essential. Opportunities for discussion should be sought and a sound knowledge of the level of tests used at dressage and Horse Trial competitions is imperative. At all examinations, but particularly higher level ones, the examiners want to see how you would teach at home; it is not wise to teach or say the things that you think the BHS wants you to say. The BHS wants competent, knowledgeable teachers who have a solid base with firm classical principles.

Protocol

Following the dressage teaching the candidate is required to give a commentary on the way that the other horse in the school is working, with special reference to the quality and purity of the paces, its way of going and its readiness to compete at medium level dressage. As the time allowed for this is only five minutes, all the candidate can do is give a snapshot of the combination. If during your teaching session you have noticed the other horse be sure to make a mental note and use the information in discussion.

Jump teaching

Again the time allowed for jump teaching is 40 minutes. An assessment should be made in the same way as in the Intermediate exam. The aim is to train the horse and rider towards Foxhunter competitions but the pupil's individual needs must always be paramount. The candidate is expected to be able to evaluate the horse's technique and should have clear ideas on how that technique can be enhanced. The candidate can ride the horse, if the rider agrees, to help with the assessment. Just as in the Intermediate exam care must be taken that the lesson is progressive. If substantial flatwork is needed, discuss this with the pupil and the examiner but some jumping work should be done. Throughout the lesson keep safety a priority and take account of other horses in the area at the same time. If the assessment of the horse has not been shared with the examiner, you will be asked to comment on the other horse and rider at the end of your lesson. As with the dressage lesson, time to study and strengthen your knowledge is essential. The expertise of the jumping teacher must be equal to that of the dressage, and on no account should the jumping be considered to be the 'poor relation'.

As with the other exams comprehensive guidelines are available from the BHS. It cannot be overemphasized that whatever exam is being worked for, the principles of teaching should be adhered to and success is only likely when the candidate has acquired considerable practical experience.

Part III
Delving Deeper

12   Teaching and Coaching as a Career

The development of equitation

Those training and coaching riders used to be concerned mainly with their overall elegance in parades and their skill in war and hunting. The first complete book still existing is by a Greek mercenary soldier writing in the fourth century BC. Xenophon came from an enlightened culture and so encouraged gentle training based on knowledge and understanding of the horse. In one particular year Xenophon rode nearly a thousand miles on a military expedition so his horse care was well based. He noted both snaffle and curb bits but saddles were at best only a folded blanket held in place by a surcingle.

Xenophon's principles of horsemanship were clearly demonstrated by Alexander the Great. He was only twelve years old (in about 350 BC) when he saw his father's grooms struggling with a fiery stallion. Alexander took over, turned the horse to face the sun so it was no longer seeing its shadow prancing beside it, and rode the horse. Bucephalus carried him until, at the age of thirty, this great horse was mortally wounded in battle.

Later, in the period dominated by Roman culture, Virgil wrote informatively about horsemanship. Progress in equitation is mostly noted from artifacts and art. By about the sixth century AD stirrups were in use in parts of Europe, but Britain was well behind the times. King Alfred the Great instituted the post of Master of the Horse in about 900 AD and yet stirrups were not seen in Britain until the Battle of Hastings in 1066.

The changing face of warfare meant that the Age of Chivalry was based on heavily encumbered knights riding powerful horses. However, during the Crusades the knights found it hard to cope with Saracens on more agile steeds and the type of horse used for war changed again.

Equitation came out of the Dark Ages in 1550 when Frederic

Grisoni from Naples published a book on riding. The Renaissance period was a time of enlightened thinking and this book with its new ideas, was well received. Grisoni was keen on riders using their legs firmly and sensitively on the horse. Grisoni taught Cesar Fiaschi who produced Pignatelli whose Neapolitan School became the most famous of the period. Indeed the Italian School of Equitation was greatly admired throughout Europe. De Pluvinel and de la Broue, students of Pignatelli, took this knowledge, skill and style to France. At this time the Spanish School of Riding was also developing. Features of this period still included domination of the horse, and riding masters would have assistants to help in the subjugation of horses. Some work was done with the horse fastened to pillars and these pillars have been retained in the traditions of the Spanish Riding School of Vienna. During the Renaissance a single pillar was also used. Severe curb bits were the norm with a wide variety of designs. The work was all based on collection and extension was neglected.

The Neapolitan schools declined due to interstate warfare. However, the French school flourished and de la Broue became keen on starting horses with a snaffle bridle. De Pluvinel instructed King Louis XIII of France and wrote the book *L'Instruction de Roi* in 1620. This book encourages the rider to appeal to the horse's intelligence and this became a hallmark of the subsequent School of Versailles.

When Charles II was forced into exile from Britain, he took with him a great horseman called William Cavendish, later the Duke of Newcastle. Cavendish learned much in Holland and after the Restoration wrote *A General System of Horsemanship* and *A New Method to Dress Horses*. Important influences on British riding in the seventeenth century were the development of fox hunting and racing.

The eighteenth century saw further advances with greater freedom of expression. In France de la Gueriniere introduced 'shoulder-in', 'counter canter' and 'flying changes'. His classic book *École de Cavalerie* (School for Riders) was published in 1733.

In Britain the Byerley Turk, the Darley Arabian and the Godolphin Arabian launched the Thoroughbred, and Weatherbys began to record thoroughbred breeding in a stud book in 1791, the same year that the first veterinary college was founded. (Vets studied only horses into the first half of the nineteenth century.) In 1805 John Adams in his book *An Analysis of Horsemanship* described hunting in a light seat, leaning forward with the weight in the stirrups. It was a new idea and did not catch on for another hundred years!

In 1848 Le Comte d'Aure became Commandant at the cavalry

school in Saumur. He was keen on outdoor riding and jumping and so clashed with the manege riders led by Baucher. D'Aure wrote *Traite d'Équitation* (1834) which preached that outdoor and school riding were complementary. General l'Hotte, Écuyer en Chef at Saumur was able to appreciate the merits of both Baucher and d'Aure and to incorporate both into the traditions of the Cadre Noir and the French cavalry.

The great manege rider of the nineteenth century was a Londoner named James Fillis. He rode in the circus in Paris and did a lot of work from the ground. Fillis preferred thoroughbreds and sought free forward movement in collection. He wrote *Breaking and Riding* (1890) and later became Chief Instructor to the cavalry in St Petersburg. Parallel developments were taking place in the great cavalry schools of Europe. The most significant changes were in Italy where Federico Caprilli developed the forward seat for cross country riding and show jumping. This allowed the horse to use itself to best advantage when galloping and jumping. Caprilli published *Principles of Cross Country Riding* in 1901 but died only a few years later whilst still developing his technique. Fortunately his work was translated into English by Piero Santini and published as *Riding Reflections* (1932), *Forward Impulse* (1936), *The Riding Instructor* (1952) and in *The Light Horse*, the popular riding magazine.

In the early 1900s talented young cavalry officers from around the world were sent to the Italian cavalry school, Pinerolo, and its sister school, Tor di Quinto, to learn the new system and to disseminate it. The greatest of these was Paul Rodzianko who took the system back to Russia in 1907. Following the First World War Rodzianko became a refugee and taught first in England and then in Ireland. Similarly Chamberlain and West took the system to Fort Riley and changed the US cavalry. Harry Chamberlain had also studied at Saumur and was a great rider and teacher; his book on training stated that 'nothing in equitation is new' yet he certainly changed American riding over fences and in showing hunters and hacks. In parallel with Chamberlain, Lt. Col. McTaggart was the great advocate of the forward seat in Britain. His book *Mount and Man* (1925) caused great controversy. At this time the Chief Instructor at the British cavalry school at Weedon, Lt. Col. Geoffrey Brooke, also wrote books showing his acceptance of the French and Italian teaching. Similarly Col. Timmis was writing about teaching and training in Canada.

The first great book based on the experience of a civilian post-First World War riding school was written by Capt. J.E. Hance. He was the father of modern riding schools in Britain and many other countries.

Taking matters further forward Capt. Vladimir Littauer, like Rodzianko a Russian exile, developed his theories in New York. This development was set out in *Commonsense Horsemanship* (1951) and *Schooling Your Horse* (1956). In England Henry Wynmalen combined his role as a Master of Foxhounds with being Britain's leading dressage rider. His books include *Equitation* (1938), *Horse Breeding and Stud Management* (1950), *Dressage* (1953) and *The Horse in Action* (1955).

In France Yves Benoust-Gironiere, a pupil of General Decarpentry, was leading equine teaching and writing. Other landmark books of the 1950s include *Modern Show Jumping* by Count Toptani, *Dressage Riding* by Richard Watjen, *Thoughts on Riding* by Brigadier Bolton, *Riding Logic* by Museler, *Horsemanship* by Seunig and *Give Your Horse a Chance* by d'Endrody.

To select the leaders of training and the great equestrian writers of the last thirty years becomes more controversial. Only with hindsight can their merits be truly judged. However, Podajhsky, setting out the teaching of the Spanish Riding School in Vienna, stands out particularly with his book *The Riding Teacher*. Perhaps the writers of the 1930s, 1940s and 1950s took equitation through a period of great change but now with international competition and communication, it is the competitions themselves which set the standards of excellence.

The development of equitation teaching

The only formal riding schools used to be those of the elite. On the one hand aristocrats had their own riding masters to produce High School horses as an art form. This began in the Renaissance 400 years ago and continued until about 100 years ago; it is still preserved in Austria by the Spanish Riding School of Vienna and in France by the Cadre Noir at Saumur. The other formal teaching of riding was by the cavalry schools which have been in existence for about two-and-a-half-thousand years. However, modern riding as we know it today only evolved when the skills of equitation were combined with the practicalities of modern cavalry teaching and the development of the forward seat following the First World War.

Up to this time riding was taught by stud grooms and head coachmen to the aristocracy who used these skills for fox hunting and pleasure. Retired soldiers, or those on leave, taught people sufficient skills for utilitarian purposes, and race riding was taught to apprentices by trainers.

Between the two World Wars the internal combustion engine superseded the horse as a means of transport, but riding for leisure became increasingly popular and the first riding schools were created. The Institute of the Horse founded the Pony Club in 1929. Following the Second World War the Institute of the Horse boldly attempted to create a national centre of excellence at St Georges near Ascot. This venture proved too costly, depleting their funds to such an extent that in 1947 the Institute of the Horse was pleased to join with the National Horse Association of Great Britain to form the British Horse Society (BHS). The BHS redeveloped the Institute of the Horse examination system and created national standards for riding and teaching.

In 1967 the BHS moved its offices to Stoneleigh in Warwickshire and the following year set up a National Equestrian Centre. Initially a National Coach was based at the Centre but the British approach favoured a system of choice, with riders only coming together immediately prior to team competitions. However, the Centre (later called the British Equestrian Centre (BEC)) proved its value as a venue for conferences, seminars and demonstrations which unified the methods and set standards under the BHS wing. In the 1990s the BEC has been the centre of a continuing quest for excellence in riding, teaching and examining. It has also been the focus of a move by the teaching and examining fraternity within the BHS to build bridges with the training groups in the disciplines of jumping, eventing, dressage, driving, vaulting and endurance riding. In addition new links, seeking unified standards, have been made with fellow organizations in Europe and the rest of the world.

On a national scale there has been a unification of ideas and practices. In the early 1980s a working group published the *Levels of Horse Care and Management* and a *Directory of Career Training in the Horse Industry*. This group was formalized in 1987 as the Joint National Horse Education and Training Council to provide a link between the government, its training organizations and the horse industry. The National Horse Education and Training Council (NHETC) has also developed National Vocational Qualifications (NVQs) for the horse industry in accordance with government dictates. These qualifications run in parallel with other examination systems in the non-thoroughbred sector but stand alone in racing and thoroughbred studs.

The other major development in education and training in the horse industry has been education in colleges of further and higher education. Starting in 1973 Warwickshire College pioneered over the next twenty years a range of ten different examinations and courses. These have been taken up by over forty other colleges throughout the British Isles. In many cases these courses are complementary to the work of the training riding schools and many students utilize both systems. Most of these college courses contain considerable practical work in addition to theory, but it should be understood that the quality of a degree course, for example, is judged by its academic standards.

Overall, the final quarter of the twentieth century has seen a blossoming of the individual sports coach, usually specializing in one discipline. Many of these coaches are current or ex-celebrity riders famous for their prowess. Other coaches have established themselves by the consistent success of their pupils. Thus the picture is one of excellent provision, reasonable harmony and a common pursuit of riders and horses happily reaching towards their full potential.

Careers in teaching

Having decided that you want to teach, how do you go about it? Do you need to be qualified? Where are you going to train and who is going to teach you? Is there a pay structure? Is it a 'proper' job that your parents will approve of?

It is recommended that all who teach are trained and qualified to a suitable level, depending on the type of teaching being carried out. If you want to teach in a riding school, for example, you must be aware of the hours you will be required to work; most riding schools have to work hardest at the weekends, school holidays and evenings, in other words in the clients' leisure time. Riding school instructors have to be realistic about when they will be able to have time off. Most instructors also have other duties, in the office or the stable yard for instance. The hours spent teaching can vary from two to eight per day depending on the establishment. The BHS Assistant Instructors Certificate will provide sufficient depth of knowledge and practical application to teach novice riders and beginners, both adults and children. After training, the Preliminary Teaching Test is taken and, from 1996, 500 hours of teaching must take place before the attainment of the Assistant Instructors Certificate.

To teach career students and first level competitors it is recommended that the BHS Intermediate Instructor's Certificate is held. The candidate has to be 20 years of age before taking the examination.

The BHS Instructors Certificate requires considerable experience and is often required by proprietors to manage their business and to teach the higher level pupils in any of the three major disciplines, dressage, show jumping and cross country. This person is able to devise training programmes for career students and to direct other instructors.

The Fellowship of the BHS is awarded to only a small number of people. It is attained through examination with a General Fellowship for those who teach a number of disciplines and have special responsibility for the development of instructors. An alternative route is based on a single specialist area chosen from show jumping, dressage, horse trials and driving and geared towards the training of competitors and their horses.

There are also formal qualifications for those who teach vaulting; these awards have been developed in conjunction with the National Coaching Foundation and the BHS. The qualification covers all aspects of horse care and lungeing as well as the gymnastic requirements. Thus the vaulting teacher has to have a wide range of skills.

The Light Horse Harness Group has developed instructor qualifications for those who teach driving. These qualifications were developed in full consultation with the BHS Training and Education department, the British Driving Society and the Horse Driving Trials Group. Assessment is through examination by a small panel of selected experts.

The Diploma in Sports Coaching for Equestrian Skills is another route to formal qualifications. At present these are only available through the BHS for approved instructors. There may be Scottish and National Vocational Qualifications (S/NVQs) with teaching units concentrating on the planning, assessment and feedback aspects of teaching. These are useful additions to other teaching certificates.

A formal educational certificate or degree is likely to be demanded for lecturing in a college offering equestrian courses. This is sometimes offered as 'on the job training' if, for example, a BHSI certificate is already held.

Teaching in a riding school is only one aspect of a teaching career. Many young people are attracted to the idea of becoming a freelance instructor. If this is your goal then ensure that the qualification that you hold is suitable for the people that you intend to teach. Maybe you would like to teach Pony Club children? Although it is not mandatory to hold a qualification you will be more in demand if you have become certificated. There are opportunities for the young trainer, both qualified and non-qualified, who is currently coaching successful competitors. This scheme is operated through the BHS Training and Education Committee for people under the age of 25 and currently teaching competition riders. The young trainers are usually involved in one specific sector of the industry and if they are selected to take part in the scheme they are apprenticed to a leading trainer in that sector. The trainer involves the successful candidate in his/her own teaching and training programmes. No fees are payable but the young person must pay accommodation and travelling expenses.

If you aspire to coach riders for competition, for example coaching children to show ponies, there are no specific qualifications. Working under an experienced coach and studying his/her techniques and expertise is the only way to become involved and to gain the experience necessary to become employable.

College lecturers are better remunerated than the average riding teacher and this has attracted a number of people into this part of the industry. Equally there are the academically inclined riding teachers who welcome the opportunity to stretch themselves mentally. Most colleges demand a specific qualification depending on the area of expertise, for example to teach equine science you may be required to hold an equine post graduate qualification with a Certificate of Education and the BHS Stable Manager's Certificate. To teach equine business studies a degree in business studies plus an industrial qualification may be necessary.

All people who teach must be technically competent themselves. They should have studied the appropriate subjects in depth and preferably have qualifications to support this, anything from a BHSAI to a degree may well be appropriate.

It is essential when teaching anything of a practical nature that suitable insurance cover is taken out. This is vital for the freelance instructor or the livery stables owner who teaches clients on their own horses. A riding school is required by law to have public liability insurance so that any person teaching at that establishment at the behest of the proprietor is automatically covered. Teaching is defined as receiving reward for advice on how to ride a horse; however, even a housewife helping a friend could be liable, so do take care.

13   How People Learn

Modern education has fallen into a trap. Instead of building on people's good points to help them excel, the student who can do a bit of everything tends to be better catered for. Have we fallen into the same trap as far as teaching riding is concerned? The traditional methods of teaching people to ride have been handed down from the army, mainly involving groups of people being commanded through a series of exercises with corrections being shouted across the school. Riding tuition has certainly progressed from this but have we really studied teaching to ensure that the methods chosen are suitable for the pupil, the lesson subject and the situation? Teaching is a vast subject with many different and fascinating paths to explore; it is useful to start by considering how the pupil learns and how the teacher establishes the learning style.

Teaching and learning a skill

A skill is defined by the Oxford English Dictionary as 'capability of accomplishing something with precision and certainty'. It has also been referred to as 'the learned ability to bring about a predetermined end product with the maximum degree of certainty and often with the minimum amount of effort'. A skilled performance is one in which the task, whatever its nature or requirements, is able to be consistently reproduced with the physical and mental involvement at their most efficient levels, needing no extraneous effort or concentration. Thus the acquisition of a skill requires an understanding of the goals to be achieved (mental ability) and dexterity at reaching them (physical ability), doing as little as possible but as much as necessary. If the skill is complex it will require a series of actions each of which involves a skilled performance.

The actions that the skilled person has acquired and finds almost automatic, are to the beginner an entanglement of separate move-ments which require conscious effort to co-ordinate. Understanding and practice lead to the mastery of a performance, for example driving a car, which is made up of individual skills requiring their own techniques.

Before teaching a skill consider the factors affecting skill acquisi-tion:

- the pupil
- the teacher
- the environment.

Each of these is influenced by other factors, for example the pupil will be affected by:

- the motivation to learn the skill;
- aptitude or talent;
- time available;
- resources available;
- physical state, e.g. tiredness;
- mental state, e.g. anxiety;
- age;
- sex;
- degree of maturity;
- intelligence.

Each pupil is an individual and must be treated as such for the best results.

The instructor is responsible for making the best use of what the pupil can offer in the way of physical and mental ability. Interesting and clear lessons will motivate the student and enhance progression, although the progress made may be physically limited by the speed at which the student can master the techniques. The instructor must bear in mind that some students are attempting to learn a skill only up to a modest level for their own enjoyment. A competent teacher is likely to be able to raise the ceiling on this preconceived level, but to prevent the teacher's own frustration and the pupils misery it should be remembered that some pupils will not have the motivation to go as far as their aptitude would allow.

A knowledge of cognitive development is useful for the student instructor; this is the development of perception in the infant as an integral part of the process resulting in intelligence. The average child has little concept of abstract thought until the age of twelve years and many adults never reach this stage in their entire lifetime. Human performance follows a basic pattern; the five senses (and that of balance) perceive the environment and relay the information to the brain which selects those messages it considers important and processes them. On the basis of the information received together with relevant stored information, the brain makes decisions affecting future activity. These messages are passed to the motor nerves which stimulate the appropriate muscle. The conversation is continuous, the sensory nerves pick up reactions from the effect of the motor nerves and relay the information to the brain which monitors the whole activity and adapts its instructions as necessary. This is intrinsic feedback or knowledge response. Normally the message goes from the sensory nerves via the spinal cord to the brain; however, basic reflexes go from the sensory nerves to the spinal cord and immediately back to the motor nerves to initiate an instantaneous reaction. As the brain is bypassed, reflexes cannot be explained or altered by logic, they are a basic survival mechanism.

Practice does not make perfect unless it is accompanied by feedback. The instructor assists pupils by giving feedback to train them to understand and make use of the feedback from their own reactions. For example, the instructor can observe the pupil's reaction to a situation and then ask the pupil to analyse that reaction and hence learn from it (Fig. 13.1). The extrinsic feedback from the instructor must be suitable for the pupil: too high a level and too much can cause confusion or a negative response; too shallow or insufficient feedback and the pupil will not progress. Eventually the teacher should need to use less feedback as the pupil becomes more aware of the intrinsic feedback from his/her own reactions.

Feedback from the instructor is necessary as it is slow and demoralizing to learn entirely by trial and error, and beginners may not always pick up the correct priorities or monitor their work adequately. They need guidance from their teachers.

Full intrinsic feedback indicates the mastery not only of understanding and practice, but also of anticipation and 'feel' – apparent intuition as to whether the action is right or wrong, and why, before it is even taken. The intuitive recognition comes from the feedback loops (sensory nerves – brain – motor nerves – carry out task – sensory nerves – brain – motor nerves – adapt task) being so well used that the task no longer requires conscious thought and co-ordination. One of

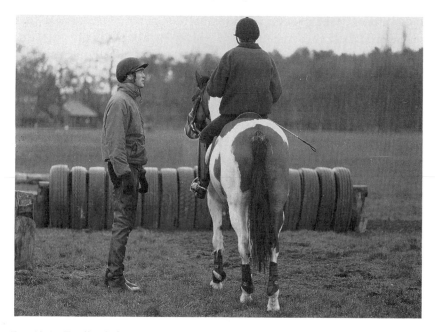

Fig. 13.1 Feedback from the teacher enhances the learning process.

the reasons why experts may not be able to pass on their own skills is that they may not remember how they do it!

Teaching based on learning

It has been suggested that real teaching only takes place if someone learns. Our knowledge of how people learn can be used to build up more effective teaching and training programmes. The acquisition of a skill can be broken down into three stages:

(1) the early cognitive phase – thinking about the task and understanding the aim by demonstration and explanation;
(2) the intermediate associative phase – practising to build up the feedback loops;
(3) the development phase – where the pupil has acquired the skill.

The 'thinking' phase involves the pupil thinking about the lesson content, the student conceptualizes the skill and is encouraged to talk through the skill with the teacher. The 'practice' phase is when the pupil tries out the new skill. During the 'development' phase the pupil becomes competent, mastering the 'feedback loops'.

To help the pupil learn, teaching the skill should be divided into manageable parts:

(1) The skill is demonstrated (Fig. 13.2).
(2) The skill is broken down into stages and the teaching points explained to the student, keeping each stage relevant to the final goal.
(3) The student talks through the skill to complete the thinking phase.
(4) The student practises the skill, with supervision to ensure feedback and the development of confidence and competence.

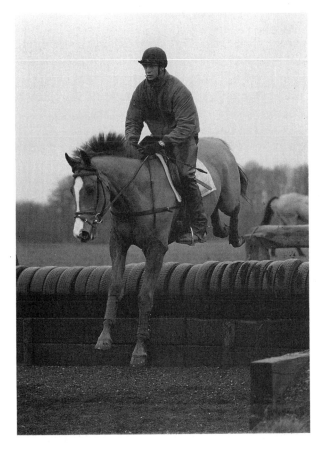

Fig. 13.2 Demonstration can help the pupil conceptualize the skill.

Usually progression is in a series of steps, so it is important to reassure the pupil, who is learning a complex skill, that he/she is nearing the ultimate goal. This is done by making the progression logical and giving a number of short term goals to promote the sense of achievement which in turn will motivate the pupil.

(5) The student evaluates his/her progress and the teacher is given the opportunity to highlight difficulties and to suggest solutions.

Remember that the way you present something to be learned will directly influence the learning skills developed by your pupils (Table 13.1).

The German author Wilhelm Museler opens the book *Riding Logic* with the words, 'Anyone can learn to ride, for riding is no more than a skill'. Riding however differs from many skills in that the pupil is dealing with another being and the horse is ruled by instincts which may seem illogical to the pupil. For example, the horse will run away if pain is caused by the rider pulling on the reins to stop him, because in the wild, flight is almost his only defence. The rider sees this as illogical because he/she knows that the pain would stop if the horse would stop. We must examine what we know of the horse's thought processes. The horse is incapable of abstract thought and relies on training to answer the rider's demands. If he is confused or frightened his first reaction is to flee and if prevented he may resort to fighting with teeth and heels.

The basic difficulty with training riders is that the horse is not constant, the reaction to the rider's signals is never exactly the same twice running, and may vary widely. The skilled rider who can produce consistent performance from a horse must have mastered his/her reactions to the intrinsic feedback received from the horse – in equine terms anticipation and feel allow the rider to vary the timing and intensity of the aids to obtain the required performance. Extrinsic feedback under these conditions requires a special skill of its own; teachers must be able to observe the smallest variations in the horse's performance and 'translate' these so that they can explain to the rider what he/she is now feeling, how to change it and what he/she should be feeling in order to enable the rider to enhance the performance of the horse.

The horse's inconsistency is partly because, unlike people, the horse cannot have his learning of a skill neatly divided into training and performance. The horse learns by trial and error and it is a measure of how quickly horses learn, that a talented horse with a talented trained

Table 13.1 Some do's and don'ts for teaching pupils.

Do	By
show that all your pupils have a contribution to make	making sure that you take notice of their views
make them seek help when they need it	not rushing in with help too soon
encourage pupils to identify and correct their own mistakes	discussion and suggested modifications to methodology
allow them time to work something out for themselves	giving them thinking time
develop their interest in learning to do things for themselves	discussing how they intend to go about learning something
develop their awareness of how to assess what they have done	checking their own work and assessing it for quality
make them realize that practice is necessary to consolidate learning and to acquire skill	encouraging them to repeat things and giving careful attention to any mistakes made

Don't	By
always make things too easy	doing the difficult bits for them, e.g. riding the horse to make it easier
do it for them when they ask for help, but encourage them to work it out for themselves	giving clues or hints
make the learning too easy	breaking it into small parts. Get them to break it up for themselves
give unrealistic feedback	giving undue praise or over-critical comment
belittle their attempts at learning	laughing at them or comparing them unfavourably with others
give tasks that are too hard or too easy	not selecting a task which is not appropriate to their previous experience

rider can reach Olympic standard in three years, while a talented but untrained rider can take two or three times as long and is likely to ruin several talented horses on the way! With the horse, training and performance are closely related; he learns by repetition so that each time he is ridden the horse is undergoing training as well as performing. This training may back up what he already knows when ridden by the accomplished rider, or sow the seeds of disobedience and incorrect work when ridden by the inadequate rider. This explains the deterioration of horses consistently ridden by novices.

Despite the many differing schools of thought about riding, everything outlined in this book applies, and those that reach Rome, by whatever road, are using remarkably similar basic methods. Indeed the similarities are far more marked than the differences in their techniques. By whatever school of thought riders are taught, those that are successful in the long term train their horses by a progressive series of gymnastic exercises over a long period. This also applies to the rider; stiff and uncoordinated riders will never reach their full potential. However well developed the feedback loops of the horse and rider, physical inability to carry out the skill will only lead to soreness and evasion.

Teaching the rider may be broken down into three phases:

(1) becoming secure;
(2) going with the horse without interfering as he performs exercises;
(3) becoming sufficiently tactful and effective to produce the performance required.

To keep these phases in the correct order the novice should learn on a generous horse which will co-operate with the clumsy and vague aids of the novice rider. Beyond the most basic level the phases are closely interrelated, as the rider cannot achieve the first two phases if the horse cannot perform the exercise. Putting the rider on the lunge will help the rider to become secure and to go with the horse without interfering as he performs exercises. However, most pupils want to ride a horse with a small amount of security at a relatively straight-forward level. Even the most dedicated are unlikely to go to the lengths of the Spanish Riding School of Vienna, where pupils remain on the lunge for three years to prevent inadequate riders causing deterioration of the horses. This time on the lunge promotes a deep seat and supple back. This independent seat will remain softly in contact with the saddle throughout any movement of the horse without any need to tighten the rest of the body – especially the legs and hands. These are the major means of communication with the horse and once tense they cannot communicate effectively. A novice rider is insufficiently independent in his/her seat to prevent the breakdown/loss of communication with momentary losses of balance.

The development of the novice into the skilled rider can be

monitored by the reactions of the horse. The less the onlooker is able to see any signals from the rider, the more the rider has developed an independent seat and intrinsic feel. Clumsiness is eliminated and the signals are so clear that they need only be very slight – the ideal of 'invisible signals', denoting the trust of the horse in the rider. The horse likes to feel that his rider is an expert. The onlooker should see only the tip of the iceberg of understanding that has gone into the acquisition of that skill.

Remember that teaching and learning are not just about giving and following a series of instructions. One person may interpret a set of instructions in a different way to another and therefore confusion could arise.

Memory

In order for people to learn they must remember what they have been taught. The memory system can be divided into three stages, each of which has a different time span:

(1) sensory memory;
(2) short term memory; and
(3) long term memory.

Sensory memory holds information for a very short period of time. This includes information that your five senses continuously gather from your immediate surroundings. If you need to retain this information it has to be transferred to the short term memory. Short term memory retains a piece of information for as long as you think about it; once you stop repeating the information to yourself you will forget it in about 20 seconds. For instance you use short term memory when you look up a phone number and repeat it to yourself until you dial the number. Some information will pass into long term memory. Long term memory holds everything from recent information to all the memories of your past, some of the information will have been deliberately memorized, some will need merely thinking about or experiencing to enter the long term memory.

Recall pattern
Recall rises for a short time after learning while the brain is sorting out

the new information and creating links between the old and new material. After that, 80% of the new detail is forgotten within 24 hours. If recall is to be kept at a reasonable level learning periods should be kept to 30 to 45 minutes. Before each break the new material should be summarized or reviewed in order for it to be retained. A break of five minutes may be adequate.

Storing information

Revision is critical in order to pass the information into the long term memory. If revision is carried out properly you can keep a high level of recall. The following revision pattern has been suggested:

- ten minutes after the learning session do ten minutes of revision; in other words, go through the work and identify essential key points and key words. For example, each lecture session should be followed by a ten minute slot in which the pupil revises the content of the lecture or lesson.
- The next day the pupil should do four minutes of revision for each learning session or lecture given the previous day. This will keep recall high for one week.
- A two minute revision period after one week will keep recall high for one month.
- A further two minute revision session after one month will firmly establish the information in the long term memory and it can now be known as knowledge.

Learning theories

Learning is a very complex process which is influenced by a large number of factors. There is, however, one certainty – no two people learn in exactly the same way. Looking back on your school days there are always some teachers you liked better than others, some you learned more from, some who commanded more respect. One of the problems that any teacher meets is that the way the pupil likes to learn is not always the same as the way the teacher likes or has been taught to teach. Ideally the teacher should be able to adapt the way that he/she teaches to fit the requirements of the pupil. This is not easy and helps to explain why one person prefers one trainer while another person cannot get on with him/her. Memory, or being able to recall what has been learned, is a vital part of the learning process.

There are several theories about the way that we learn, including:

- the analytical and creative role of the left and right sides of the brain;
- personal styles;
- neuro-linguistic programming.

Analytical and creative talents

Intelligence or the ability to analyse and organize facts is necessary for effective learning. Intelligent people are usually articulate. Creativity and the ability to come up with new ideas is less likely to be expressed in words and consequently has been given less status than intelligence.

The brain consists of two parts each with its own particular functions. Broadly speaking the left of the brain (which controls the right side of the body) is associated with intelligence and the right side of the brain (which controls the left side of the body) with creativity. If the left side of the brain is dominant the person is likely to be logical and analytical, preferring step-by-step learning with verbal explanations. A more 'right-brained' person is likely to be creative and intuitive, preferring holistic learning with visual explanations. Traditional methods of teaching encourage left brain learning, emphasizing analytical thinking, and are rewarded, for example, by the attainment of written examinations. By not using both sides of the brain we are halving our potential, but we can develop that side of the brain that has been neglected.

As teachers we need to be aware of our own preferred style of learning so that we can modify it to suit the preferred style of the pupil. A left-brained analytical jumping trainer who is fascinated with the intricacies of every element of the horse's way of going is unlikely to inspire a right-brained intuitive pupil who is interested only in jumping clear rounds. Similarly the right-brained creative trainer is likely to frustrate the left-brained pupil who wants to understand each step before proceeding to the next.

The best teachers are those who have a holistic approach, using both sides of the brain, and are able to look at the broad picture, consider the implications of their actions and to stimulate and collect good ideas from many people. Inspiration comes from the right brain; the ability to analyse and translate those ideas into action comes from the left brain. Following Table 13.2, mark yourself on a scale of one to five to identify if you use more right or left brain or both equally.

Table 13.2 Left brain/right brain.

		Left brain	Right brain
(1)	Do you remember most easily	the words of a song? names?	the tune of a song? faces?
(2)	When learning something new, do you prefer	verbal description? abstract concepts? each step fully explained? to read about how something works?	diagrams/illustrations? concrete examples? an overall picture first? to find out by manipulating it?
(3)	Which do you work with more easily?	mathematical formulae? multiple choice questions? step-by-step checking? thoughts?	forms and patterns? open-ended questions? inspired guesswork? feelings?
(4)	How would you describe yourself?	methodical? analytical? logical?	spontaneous? creative? imaginative?

Personality and learning styles

In the 1970s David Kolb developed a theory of how people learn. As soon as they are born people start to take in information and this continues throughout life. Combined with the active process of problem-solving all this information is stored as experience. People use their experience to build the concepts, rules and principles which guide them in new situations. As a person's experience of life expands, these concepts are modified to make them more effective. This happens in a four-stage cycle as shown in Fig. 13.3.

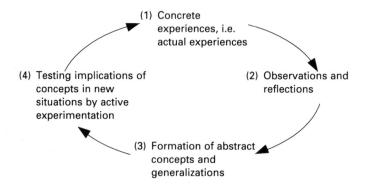

Fig. 13.3 The four-stage cycle of learning.

This learning cycle takes place constantly, with our needs and goals determining what we learn most readily. We perceive goals, seek related experiences, interpret the experiences in the light of our goals, form concepts from them and test the implications. If the goals are not clear, learning is erratic and inefficient. Depending on their personality people develop a learning style which may emphasize one part of the learning cycle at the expense of another. For example, we may accept experiences but fail to learn from them as not enough time is spent on observation and reflection.

Identifying your learning style

Look at the pairs of words in Table 13.3 and choose the one that best describes your behaviour. Tick columns A or D if you strongly identify with the concept or tick columns B or C to indicate a slight preference. Do the same for the pairs of words in Table 13.4, marked 1 to 4.

Table 13.3   Identifying your learning style (1).

	A	B	C	D	
Talks to					Listens to
Makes suggestions					Gives a critique
Finds solutions					Identifies problems
Experiments					Digests
Doing					Considering
Answers questions					Asks questions
Improvises					Plans
Impatient					Cautious
Goes step-by-step					Wants the whole picture
Up-and-about					Sits and thinks
Total					

Circle your highest score from A to D and 1 to 4 and enter them on the grid (Fig. 13.4). Draw a line down the box under your highest letter, A to D. Draw a line across the box from your highest number, 1 to 4. Where the lines intersect indicates your personality style. If you have two equal scores for the letters and/or lines, enter lines for both. This indicates that you use two primary learning styles and have a range of behaviour. If you have a strong second, plot that also. If you score in the corners it indicates that you identify very strongly with that learning style.

Table 13.4 Identifying your learning style (2).

	1	2	3	4	
Personal					Impersonal
Uses gut feeling and hunches					Relies on fact and reason
Discusses with others					Analyses alone
Interested in people					Interested in things
Concerned with effect					Concerned with design
Looks for new experiences					Looks for new ideas
Works sporadically					Works to a timetable
Impulsive					Methodical
Ruled by heart					Ruled by head
Total					

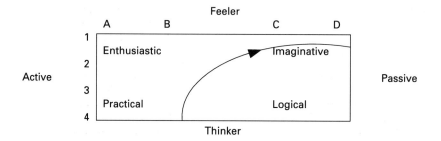

Fig. 13.4 Identifying your learning style (3).

The teacher needs to create the idea, work out the teaching plan and then teach it (Fig. 13.5). In other words he/she needs to possess parts of all four learning styles that we have identified.

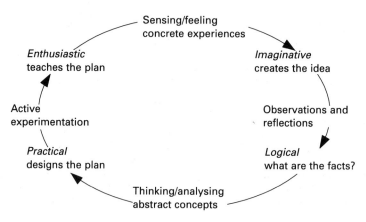

Fig. 13.5 Teaching using all four learning styles.

Table 13.5 Characteristics of each personality style.

Enthusiastic (feeling and doing)	*Imaginative (feeling and taking in)*
• likes to get involved	• avoids interfering or challenging
• shares ideas, tells others	• uses insight, dreams
• thrives on new situations	• listens to others
• open-minded, not sceptical	• unhurried, casual, friendly
• sometimes seen as pushy	• observes, asks questions
• consults lots of people	• watches with fascination
• operates on a trial and error gut reaction basis	• works in occasional bursts of energy, not much contemplation
• likes to discharge emotion	• picks up on feelings
• wants to make things happen	• sees the whole picture
• responds immediately	• backs off from pressure

Practical (doing and thinking)	*Logical (taking in and thinking)*
• absorbed by practical problems	• likes theories and ideas
• tries out ideas to see if they work	• makes new models in head
• wants to get on with things	• precise, thorough, careful
• impatient with 'too much talk'	• likes to think things through first
• gets things done	• organizes and plans
• uses factual data	• sceptical
• good detective skills	• calculates the probabilities
• loses sight of the context	• notices the pitfalls
• little awareness of others	• reacts slowly, wants facts
• likes to be in control	• can be dogmatic
• poor at getting on with others	• blocks things getting done

Table 13.6 Advantages of each learning style.

Enthusiastic	*Imaginative*
• gets totally involved in things that interest/are interesting	• sees new ways to do things
• enjoys writing freely	• invents creative solutions
• asks for help, talks through problems and is not concerned with appearing silly	• sees long term implications
• doesn't get in a flap	
• presents work in novel way	
• often reaches accurate conclusions in absence of logical justification	• sees connections between areas being studied
	• pinpoints new questions

Practical	*Logical*
• works well alone	• organizes facts and material
• good at setting goals and making plans of action	• enjoys theoretical problems
• reads instructions carefully	• prioritizes work
• gets things done on time	• reworks essays and notes
• classifies and files notes	• needs minimum help from teachers
• sees the application of theory	• likes to understand everything
• methodical	• precise and thorough
	• a good critic

Table 13.7 Disadvantages of each learning style.

Enthusiast	*Imaginative*
● doesn't plan work ● tries to do too many things at once ● can be demanding of friends ● leaves things until the last minute ● doesn't check work or redo ● can't be bothered with details ● drops things easily, changes tack	● forgets important details ● waits too long before getting started ● only works when in the mood ● forgets to bring important books, etc. ● won't stick to timetables ● too easy going, not assertive enough
Practical	*Logical*
● doesn't question basic concepts ● impatient with others' views ● thinks that theirs is the only way ● more concerned with getting the job done than doing it well ● doesn't work well with others ● not interested in presentation	● only trusts logic ● gets bogged down in theory ● reluctant to try new approaches ● needs too much information before getting started ● misses opportunities ● won't ask for help ● poor in group discussion

Once the personality style has been identified teachers need to consider how their teaching style should be modified to suit the needs of other types of learners.

Practical
Practicalists learn best from activities where:

● they are given techniques currently applicable to their jobs;
● they are given immediate opportunities to implement what they have learned;
● they can deal with 'real' problems;
● they can concentrate on practical issues;
● there is an obvious link between the subject matter and a problem or opportunity in practice.

They learn least when:

● learning is not related to immediate needs;
● learning is all theory and general principles;
● there is no practice or clear guidelines on how to do it;
● there is no apparent reward from learning – it does not apply to the here and now.

Imaginative
Imaginatives learn best where:

- they are allowed to watch and think;
- they can stand back and listen;
- they are allowed to think before acting;
- they can reach a decision in their own time without pressure and deadlines.

Imaginatives learn least when:

- they are 'forced' to act as a leader or spokesman;
- they have to do something without warning;
- they are given dogmatic instructions about how things should be done;
- they are not given sufficient information from which to draw conclusions.

Logical
Logics learn best where:

- they have time to explore the facts methodically;
- they can listen or read about rational ideas and concepts;
- they have to understand complex situations;
- the situation is structured with a clear purpose.

They learn least when:

- the situation involves emotions or feelings;
- they have to do something out of context or without reason;
- they find the subject shallow or gimmicky;
- they feel out of place, e.g. working with enthusiasts or imaginatives.

Enthusiasts
Enthusiasts learn best where:

- there are new experiences and opportunities;
- there is excitement and a range of diverse activities;
- they are involved with other people;
- they have a high profile, e.g. leading groups.

They learn least when:

- learning is passive, e.g. lectures;
- they are asked to stand back and not get involved;
- they have to learn 'theoretical' material;
- they have to repeat, e.g. practising a skill.

Most people are a mixture of each of these learning styles; identifying their major influences is very useful when teaching on a one-to-one basis but can prove more difficult in group teaching.

Neuro-linguistic Programming (NLP)

Neuro-linguistic Programming (NLP) is based on the study of the behaviour of successful people and assumes that what and how we think is based on the immediate input of the five senses. Thinking affects the way our body works and is particularly reflected in facial movement and expression. It is said that what you are thinking can be picked up from the way you move your eyes. People have preferred communication styles based on hearing, seeing and feeling. Their preference is likely to affect the way they learn. The three main forms of communication are:

- visual – prefers to see things than talk about them and thinks in pictures. People who operate in the visual mode need to see what is meant and are often imaginative. They may respond better to explanations that are diagrammatic rather than spoken.
- auditory – prefers to hear presentations and talk out problems. This relies on verbal communication and is the mode used by the traditional education system.
- kinaesthetic – prefers to be involved, active, moving. This is the primary mode for music, dancing and sport and involves moving and feeling. Those who operate in the kinetic mode are often reluctant to talk but quick to pick up on feelings.

Visual learners typically say 'I see now', 'That looks right to me', 'I need to get it into perspective'. Auditory learners may say 'That sounds right', 'Suddenly it clicked', 'I can hear that you are unhappy'. Kinaesthetic learners will say 'That feels right', 'I find it difficult to handle', 'Give me an example'. By matching the teaching approach to the learner you can communicate more effectively.

Our society recognizes the intellectual mode above the others; logic and reason are valued and we are taught to be objective and not emotional. Teaching sport, including riding, which is essentially kinetic sometimes focuses more upon the learning techniques of watch and listen, whereas it should concentrate on 'getting the feel for it'. Teaching is often so much restricted to telling that we have lost the instinct to help learning by using visual and kinetic modes.

Teaching the rider

We have already identified that there are several different learning styles. As far as the riding teacher is concerned, people essentially fall into two main groups: activists and theorists. Activists are practical people, they would like a lesson to be primarily a 'doing' lesson but it is also beneficial to these people to learn to think and evaluate. Similarly the theorists need to be encouraged to put their thoughts into action and then evaluate the outcome. Most class rides combine these two styles of learning and the following scenario may well illustrate how the problem of learning styles and mixed abilities within a group might be overcome.

A riding club has the following group assembled for a 'one-off' lesson:

Sue: a theorist with a six-year-old show hunter which is quite green.
Pat: an activist with a nine-year-old elementary dressage champion which gets bored easily.
Deirdre: an activist with a ten-year-old horse working at medium level with a hot temperament.
Tim: an activist with a six-year-old Irish Draught horse that is lazy and green.
Sarah: a theorist/activist with an eight-year-old all rounder with a rather keen temperament.
Hazel: a theorist/activist with a fourteen-year-old intermediate eventer which is stiff and unresponsive.

At first sight these riders and horses appear to have little in common and it is hard to find a common theme which would result in a satisfactory lesson plan. However, on closer investigation it can be seen that all horses are, in one way or another, not responsive to the aids. What exercise improves the responsiveness to the aids? The best is 'transitions'. We have a mixed ability group so the transitions must be practised so that all participants gain from the session. For example, Sue would be asked to start with 'walk–trot' transitions and move on to 'trot–halt' transitions which are allowed to be progressive but of a quality that demands that the horse steps under and does not resist the bit. On the other hand, Pat would be asked to go directly from 'halt–trot, trot–halt' with accuracy, impulsion and swing. This would help Pat's horse to become lighter in front and with a better self carriage.

There will be shades between which would help all the group and the session can progress to canter transitions, up and down, and also to transitions within the paces. At the end of the lesson, Sue, the theorist, could be invited to lead evaluation and feedback discussions in order to encourage Tim, an activist, to begin to think a little more about his horse's way of going, rather than simply relying on 'feel'.

14   Giving a Lecture

People frequently find public speaking very intimidating and while many riding teachers are quite at home in a practical environment, standing up in front of a group of students and delivering a lecture can be daunting. Lecturing, like any other skill, requires practice. The more thought and planning that goes into a lecture, the better it will be and the more confident the lecturer will be when delivering the material. It is useful to consider the subject under several headings:

- lecture planning
- the lecture room
- preparing a lecture
- lecture presentation
- use of equipment
- improving lecturing technique.

Planning

Your audience will appreciate a commonsense approach and a logical development of ideas throughout the lecture. Adequate and careful preparation is essential. The material required for the lecture should be gathered together, the script of the lecture written out and read through several times. This ensures that the lecturer is familiar with the content, and although you are not trying to memorize the script, the subject will be firmly placed in your subconscious, allowing you to be confident.

The next step is to condense the script of the lecture into main headings which can be written in large letters on cards. If you know the content of the lecture, a glance at the heading will prompt you to remember the content relevant to that heading. If figures, quotes or complex words are involved these can also be written on the card to act as additional prompts. You must not lecture by reading your full notes; this is boring for the audience and inhibits any spontaneity.

Experienced lecturers are not tied to their notes. They allow the reaction of the audience to guide them – perhaps a certain point has not gone home and needs to be rephrased and repeated before going on to the next point. Scanning the faces of your listeners and how they are reacting will let you know if you have got your point home. Another advantage of not reading your notes is that it allows you to talk to the audience, look them straight in the face and they will feel that you are talking directly to them. This is useful in maintaining attention and discipline.

Good timing is essential; it is just as bad to run out of material as it is to fail to cover everything necessary. It is useful to allocate a maximum amount of time to be spent on each point and to write that on the prompt card. Remember to leave enough time for questions from your audience.

The lecture room

A lecture does not have to be conducted in a purpose-built lecture theatre but can be delivered very effectively in any room, provided that a little thought is given to its layout. There should be plenty of fresh air and it should not be too warm, otherwise the audience will soon be asleep! The lighting should be adequate as bad lighting makes the listener uncomfortable – do not turn the lights off to show slides and expect pupils to take notes in the dark. Make sure that you as the lecturer can be seen and heard and that you in turn can see all the audience – eye contact is very important both for maintaining discipline and for developing a rapport with your audience. Too many charts and diagrams will brighten the room up but they will also distract attention from the lecture.

Presentation

Personality plays an important part in lecture technique. Try to make it obvious that you enjoy lecturing, that you know your subject and that you are there to help. This means that you have to be confident and well prepared. Nerves afflict most lecturers at some time; try to feel that as the lecturer you are the master of the situation and that you are in charge of the direction that the lecture takes. Try not to show your nerves but, on the other hand, do not appear arrogant or over-confident. Breathe deeply and talk slowly; nerves make most people speak too rapidly. You should face your audience at all times; stop talking when you are writing information on the board or chart. Try not to fidget, and stand still; move only when you need to demonstrate a point. Nerves lead many lecturers to have mannerisms which may irritate or distract the listeners. On the other hand try not to look like a statue – be natural. Bear in mind the following points. Do not:

- look at a point over the heads of the audience;
- keep looking at your watch;
- jangle keys or money in your pocket;
- wave your arms about, fidget and pace about;
- speak in a voice that is not your own, in other words, adopt an affected accent;
- be sarcastic, get cross or raise a cheap laugh at the expense of one of the audience;
- be theoretical or bluff;
- write on the board and talk at the same time;
- swear!
- read from or make it obvious that you are referring to notes;
- use pet phrases;
- be drawn away from the point.

Do:

- stand still;
- make your point clearly by illustrations if possible;
- speak clearly and a little more slowly than normal;
- be honest – if you are asked a question that you cannot answer, say so and volunteer to find out the answer;
- take your watch off and position it by your notes so that you can keep to time discreetly;
- print clearly when you write on the board;
- use simple language that the audience will understand;
- keep to the point.

Preparation

The first thing to do is to establish what you are going to talk about. Find out the following:

- the title or subject of the lecture;
- the audience – age, number, previous experience, expectations;
- the duration;
- the location and facilities available.

The title of the talk may be very broad, such as feeding your horse. How you tackle this enormous subject will be dictated by your audience and how long you have to cover the subject. You will be able to go into detail on all aspects of feeding if you are speaking to a group of career students for ten 60-minute lectures. However, if a riding club group invites you to speak for 45 minutes at an evening meeting you will have to be both entertaining and informative about a small aspect of equine nutrition. Speak to the organizer and try to get an idea of what the audience wants; this is easy for the career student who has clear goals, such as passing an exam. It is more difficult if the group contains a variety of ages and experience. In this situation keep the information simple and find some ground that is common to all the audience, for example, give them basic guidelines for rationing so that they can apply what you say to their own horses.

Research

Having decided on the subject and the depth of coverage you then have to research the subject. Make detailed notes from a variety of sources so that you can give a balanced account, taking care that the material that you use is up-to-date. This will help you become thoroughly familiar with the subject, so that if you are questioned you will be able to answer with confidence. These notes are the background for the talk you are going to give.

Writing the talk

Go through the detailed notes and highlight the main headings or areas you want to cover in the talk. Also pick out specific facts that you feel are important. Transfer these headings onto small prompt cards. Use large print and a highlighting pen so that you can read the cards easily. The headings on the prompt cards will spark your memory so that you can speak naturally using your knowledge of the background notes.

Visual aids

As you go through the detailed notes you may identify areas that need illustration to clarify them for the audience, for example, if you are talking about the digestive system it makes sense to have a diagram of it. You can prepare visual aids as handouts for the audience to refer to as you are speaking, but this can be distracting as people shuffle their bits of paper or drop them on the floor. Alternatively you can draw the information onto a flip chart, board or acetate. Acetates are clear sheets which are put onto an overhead projector; you can either photocopy onto the acetate or write on it. Remember, all visual aids must:

- be easy to read – print boldly and use strong colours;
- not contain too much information.

Many people use an acetate with headings instead of prompt cards; a piece of paper covers the acetate and this is moved to reveal each heading in turn. Turn off the overhead projector when you are not using it – the light is distracting and it is noisy and hot. If you are pointing to information on the screen use a pencil or pointer – fingers are stubby and get in the way. Do not fall into the trap of turning your back to the audience to read the screen – you must know by heart the information on each acetate. You may choose to use a slide projector to illustrate your talk; this can be very lively and successful as people can see pictures of horses which is what really interests them. However, as soon as you dim the lights you lose the attention of your audience unless you are a very effective and experienced speaker.

Structuring the talk

The talk must have a beginning, a middle and an end, in other words an introduction, the bulk of the talk and a conclusion. Always start by greeting your audience and introducing yourself (if not already done), then introduce your subject and outline the format of the talk and what you hope to achieve. You will get the attention of the audience if they feel that there is a goal to be achieved. If it is an informal talk you may ask them to ask questions as you go along or, in more formal circumstances, you may ask them to save any questions to the end. The conclusion should consist of a summary of the points you have made, you may thank your audience for their attention and then ask if there are any questions. You may decide to consolidate your lecture by giving people a summary of its content at the end. Once the lecture is prepared you should then practise the talk and allocate time to each part or heading that you have identified; write this on your prompt card so that you can run to time.

Delivering the lecture

Make sure that you arrive in plenty of time so that you can alter the layout of the room if necessary and check any equipment you are using. Projectors and screens are notorious for going wrong at the last moment. Run through the talk in your head or read through your prompt cards so that you are tuned into your subject and then deliver your lecture with confidence. If possible be informal and approachable and allow your personality to keep the attention of your audience. If you are asked awkward questions or ones that are outside your knowledge then have the confidence to admit that you do not know and possibly throw the question open to the audience – there may be someone there who knows. If you are giving a series of lectures, find out the answer for the next session.

How to improve your lecture technique

As always you can learn from others; listen to and observe those who lecture to you and make note of the good and bad points and use these tips to develop your own lecturing style. Once you have prepared your talk, practise it so that you are at ease with the material and the timing and only have to cope with your nerves. If you find speaking to an audience difficult, develop your voice and confidence by reading aloud a passage from a book. Speak naturally using good grammar and clear enunciation and, above all, try to enjoy yourself.

Appendix 1
Exercises to Include in Lesson Plans

In order to develop the content of your lesson it is a good idea to practise lessons containing specific work. This encourages you to be detailed in your observation and gives plenty of time for pupil feedback. These exercises can form all or part of a lesson and have been divided into categories to allow you to 'pick and mix' to meet the needs of the individual or class that you are teaching.

Exercises in walk

(1) For all riders
Simple turns, circles and loops. Transitions. Small half circles paying attention to bend and rhythm. Work on a long rein to encourage free walk.
(2) Working towards 'connection' between the hand and the leg
Leg yield on circles and straight lines. Shoulder-in. Smaller circles and straight lines. Small travers. Transitions. Work on a long rein. Medium and extended walk.
(3) Working towards collection
Half pass, travers, demi-pirouettes to encourage engagement. Rein back. Transitions. Medium, collected and extended walk.

Exercises in trot

(1) For all riders
Simple turns, circles and loops. Transitions. Putting emphasis throughout on rhythm, balance and acceptance of the aids. Encouraging the horse to start to stretch.
(2) Working towards 'connection' between the hand and the leg
Leg yield on circles and straight lines. Shoulder-in. Smaller circles and

half circles. Small travers. Improving transitions. Variations within the pace.

(3) Working towards collection
Half pass, travers, shoulder-in. Transitions within the pace. Direct and progressive transitions.

Exercises in canter

(1) For all riders
Circles. Transitions trot–canter, canter–trot. Establishing rhythm, balance and acceptance of the aids.

(2) Working towards 'connection' between the leg and the hand
Loops. Simple change. Counter canter. Establishing self carriage. Variations within the pace. Keeping the horse 'in front of the leg'.

(3) Working towards collection
Developing self carriage. Half pass, travers, smaller circles. Developing counter canter. Variations within the pace. Direct and progressive transitions.

Gymnastic exercises

Trot (Fig. 1)

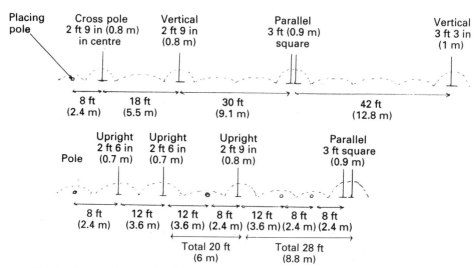

Fig. 1 Gymnastic exercises in trot.

(1) Riding in a light seat, cease rising without the seat in the saddle, adopting a poised or hover position.
(2) Work over a series of poles and raised poles set 4–5.5 ft (1.2–1.7 m) apart, both on a straight line and on a circle. Work up to six poles using rising, sitting and the poised position in trot.
(3) Build up a grid, add one component at a time and work from a different direction each day.
(4) Vary the rein contact through the grid as a balance exercise for the rider.

Canter

(1) Riding in a light seat, vary the position to establish strengths and weaknesses.
(2) Canter to a pole on the ground to enable the rider to find the rhythm and to ensure that the pole is negotiated out of this rhythm. It may be necessary to lengthen a little or to contain a little but it is vital that the rider becomes 'rhythm aware'.
(3) Add more poles 8–9 ft (2.4–2.7 m) apart and maintain balance throughout, on a straight line and a curve.
(4) Progressively build up grids.

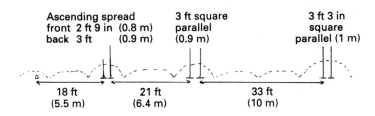

Fig. 2 Developing scope.

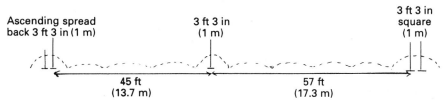

Fig. 3 Developing rhythm.

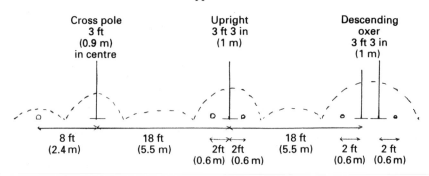

Fig. 4 Developing technique, bascule and fore leg action.

Factors that affect distances

- A horse going downhill will tend to take a longer stride.
- A horse going uphill will tend to take a shorter stride.
- Heavy going will shorten the stride.
- Ideal going may lengthen the stride.
- Towards the entrance/exit may lengthen the stride.
- Away from the entrance/exit may shorten the stride.

	Outdoors	Indoors
Three non-jumping strides	46–48 ft (14–14.6 m)	45–47 ft (13.7–14.3 m)
Four non-jumping strides	57–60 ft (17.3–18.3 m)	56–59 ft (17–18 m)
Five non-jumping strides	68–72 ft (20.7–21.9 m)	67–71 ft (20.4–21.6 m)

Fig. 5 Suggested distances for a related stride (show jumping).

Figures 6–9 suggest minimum and maximum distances to be used in open combinations on level ground in normal weather conditions. For novice competitions (3 ft 5 in–3 ft 9 in, 1–1.1 m) the shorter distances should be used. Above 3 ft 9 in (1.1 m) the distances may be lengthened. In treble combinations both distances must be consistent. Indoors up to 6 in (15 cm) for one stride and 12 in (30 cm) for two strides may be deducted from the distances.

Figure 10 suggests minimum and maximum distances for 14.2 hh (148 cm) ponies. For 13.2 hh (138 cm) ponies, 1 ft 6 in (0.4 m) should be deducted for a one stride distance and 2 ft (0.6 m) for a two stride distance. For 12.2 hh (128 cm) ponies, 3 ft (0.9 m) should be deducted

		upright	true parallel	ascending oxer
upright	(1 stride) (Fig. 7) (2 strides)	24–26 ft (7.3–7.9 m) 34 ft 6 in–36 ft (10.5–11 m)	23 ft 6 in–25 ft (10.5–10.8 m) 34 ft 6 in–35 ft 6 in (10.5–10.8 m)	23–25 ft (7–7.6 m) 34 ft–35 ft 6 in (10.3–10.8 m)
true parallel	(1 stride) (Fig. 8) (2 strides)	24 ft 6 in–25 ft 6 in (7.4–7.7 m) 34 ft 6 in–35 ft 6 in (10.5–10.8 m)	23–24 ft (7–7.3 m) 34–35 ft (10.3–10.6 m)	22 ft 6 in–24 ft (6.8–7.3 m) 33–35 ft (10–10.6 m)
ascending oxer	(1 stride) (Fig. 9) (2 strides)	24 ft 6 in–26 ft (7.4–7.9 m) 34 ft 6 in–36 ft (10.5–11 m)	23–24 ft 6 in (7–7.4 m) 34–35 ft 6 in (10.3–10.8 m)	22 ft 6 in–24 ft 6 in (6.8–7.4 m) 33 ft 6 in–35 ft 6 in (10.2–10.8 m)

Fig. 6 Suggested distances for show jumping (horses).

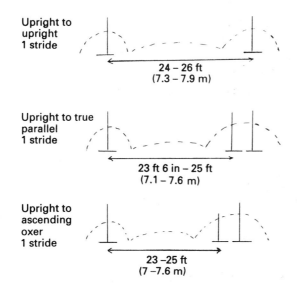

Fig. 7

for a one stride distance and 3 ft 11 in (1.2 m) for a two stride distance.

The suggested distances in Fig. 12 are for combination fences cross country. They are total lengths, including take off and landing and could be found when competing at novice (3 ft 6 in, 1.07 m) to Advanced (3 ft 11 in, 1.2 m).

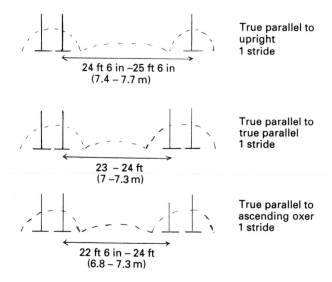

24 ft 6 in –25 ft 6 in
(7.4 – 7.7 m)

True parallel to
upright
1 stride

23 – 24 ft
(7 –7.3 m)

True parallel to
true parallel
1 stride

22 ft 6 in – 24 ft
(6.8 – 7.3 m)

True parallel to
ascending oxer
1 stride

Fig. 8

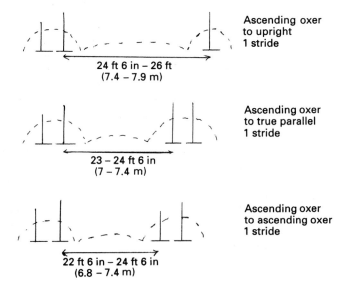

24 ft 6 in – 26 ft
(7.4 – 7.9 m)

Ascending oxer
to upright
1 stride

23 – 24 ft 6 in
(7 – 7.4 m)

Ascending oxer
to true parallel
1 stride

22 ft 6 in – 24 ft 6 in
(6.8 – 7.4 m)

Ascending oxer
to ascending oxer
1 stride

Fig. 9

		upright	true parallel	ascending oxer
upright	(1 stride)	22–24 ft 6 in (6.7–7.4 m)	22–23 ft 6 in (6.7–7.1 m)	22–23 ft 6 in (6.7–7.1 m)
	(2 strides)	32–34 ft 6 in (9.7–10.5 m)	31 ft 6 in–33 ft 6 in (9.6–10.2 m)	31 ft 6 in–33 ft 6 in (9.6–10.2 m)
true parallel	(1 stride)	22–24 ft 6 in (6.7–7.4 m)	22–23 ft (6.7–7 m)	22–23 ft (6.7–7 m)
	(2 strides)	32–34 ft 6 in (9.7–10.5 m)	31–32 ft 6 in (9.4–9.9 m)	31–32 ft 6 in (9.45–9.9 m)
ascending oxer	(1 stride)	22–24 ft 6 in (6.7–7.4 m)	22–23 ft (6.7–7 m)	22–23 ft (6.7–7 m)
	(2 strides)	32–34 ft 6 in (9.7–10.5 m)	31–33 ft (9.4–10 m)	31–33 ft (9.45–10 m)

Fig. 10 Suggested distances for show jumping (ponies).

Number of strides	Minimum distances	Maximum distances
Bounce	12 ft (3.6 m)	15 ft (4.5 m)
1	18 ft (5.5 m)	28 ft (8.5 m)
2	30 ft (9.1 m)	39 ft (11.9 m)
3	45 ft (13.7 m)	52 ft (15.8 m)
4	54 ft (16.4 m)	64 ft (19.5 m)
5	69 ft (21 m)	78 ft (23.8 m)
6	81 ft (24.7 m)	91 ft (27.7 m)

Fig. 11 Suggested distances for a related stride (cross country).

	Bounce	1 stride	2 strides
Upright to upright	12–15 ft (3.6–4.5 m)	24–27 ft (7.3–8.2 m)	35–38 ft (10.6–11.6 m)
Upright to parallel or parallel to upright	12–14 ft (3.6–4.2 m)	24–26 ft (7.3–7.9 m)	33–36 ft (10–11 m)
Parallel to parallel	(not recommended)	24–26 ft (7.3–7.9 m)	33–36 ft (10–11 m)
Step up and down	9 ft (2.7 m)	18 ft (5.5 m)	—
Rails to step up	8 ft	21–24 ft (6.4–7.3 m)	—
Rails to step down	8 ft	18–21 ft (5.5–6.4 m)	—

Fig. 12 Suggested distances in combination fences cross country.

	Bounce	1 stride	2 strides
Step up to rails	9 ft (2.7 m)	18–20 ft (5.5–6.1 m)	—
Step down to rails	10–12 ft (3–3.6 m)	18–21 ft (5.5–6.4 m)	—
Coffins			
on easy slope	—	18–20 ft (5.5–6.1 m)	—
on difficult slope	—	15 ft (4.5 m) up 16–18 ft (4.9–5.5 m) down	
Ditch and rails	9–12 ft (2.7–3.6 m)	18–20 ft (5.5–6.1 m)	—

Fig. 12 Continued.

Appendix 2
The International Code of Conduct

(1) In all equestrian sports the welfare of the horse must be considered paramount.

(2) The well-being of the horse shall take precedence over the demands of breeders, trainers, riders, drivers, owners, dealers, organizers, sponsors, officials and other commercial interests.

(3) All handling and veterinary treatment must ensure the health and welfare of the horse.

(4) The highest standards of nutrition, health, sanitation and safety shall be encouraged and maintained at all times.

(5) Adequate provision must be made for ventilation, feeding, watering and maintaining a healthy environment during travelling.

(6) Emphasis should be placed on increasing education in training and equestrian practices and on promoting scientific studies in equine health.

(7) In the interests of the horse, the fitness and competence of the rider or driver shall be regarded as essential.

(8) All training methods should take account of the horse as a living creature and must not include any technique considered by the Federation Equestre Internationale (FEI) to be abusive.

(9) National Federations must establish adequate controls in order that all persons and bodies under their jurisdiction respect the welfare of the horse.

(10) Rules regarding the health and welfare of horses must be strictly adhered to, not only in competition, but also in training. Such rules and regulations shall be regularly reviewed.

Explanatory notes

(1) In all equestrian sports the welfare of the horse must be considered paramount.

At every level of equestrian sport there are pressures on owners, competitors, trainers and grooms in the preparation of horses and ponies for events and at the competition itself. Sometimes these pressures are conflicting. Usually it is quite clear what is in the best interest of the horse and what is not. It is essential that the welfare of the horse is considered above all else.

(2) The well-being of the horse shall take precedence over the demands of breeders, trainers, riders, drivers, owners, dealers, organizers, sponsors, officials and other commercial interests.

There are times when performance in a competition may need to come second to the well-being of the horse. For example, in our modern world when commercial interest can come above all else, there could be a temptation to push a horse beyond its capabilities. This must be resisted at all costs. Organizers and officials have a particular responsibility to avoid situations whereby a horse could be exploited and should make sponsors aware that such dangers exist.

(3) All handling and veterinary treatment must ensure the health and welfare of the horse.

The person responsible for the horse must ensure that all who handle it are competent. Where treatment other than first aid is required a veterinarian should be consulted. The pressures to compete can lead to abuse of the horses or the use of practices prohibited by the FEI.

(4) The highest standards of nutrition, health, sanitation and safety shall be encouraged and maintained at all times.

Both at home and at events the person responsible for the horse must ensure that its living conditions are of the highest possible standard. The provision of good quality feed and a clean plentiful water supply is mandatory. The stable should be well ventilated and hygiene and sanitary conditions must be carefully monitored to ensure that there is minimal risk of infection or disease. At events this is the responsibility of the organizing committee. Although it is also the organizers' responsibility to set safety standards at events, ultimately it is up to the person responsible for the horse to ensure its safety.

(5) Adequate provision must be made for ventilation, feeding, watering and maintaining a healthy environment during travelling.

Care in ensuring that horses to be transported are free from even minor respiratory or other disease is essential to their well-being. Attention to the provision of adequate ventilation at all times, but particularly when motor vehicles or aircraft carrying horses are stationary for long periods, will help to minimize equine transit stress. Changes in temperature and moisture content of air breathed by horses in transit are almost inevitable during the transport process. Water should be offered every six to eight hours from the start of the journey whether by road or air, and if hay is to be made available to reduce transit-associated weight loss, it should be clean and as free as possible from fungal contamination.

Undue delays must be avoided and overnight rest periods should be arranged where appropriate. The protection of the horse and the maintenance of an ambient temperature are essential factors to be considered throughout the journey. A driver of horse transport vehicles should take into account the safety and comfort of the horse. Rectal temperature should be recorded twice a day for a few days after arrival, following long journeys. Monitoring bodyweight may be helpful in the post transit management of horses.

(6) Emphasis should be placed on increasing education in training and equestrian practices and on promoting scientific studies in equine health.

National Federations are responsible for providing training and education in all aspects of horse care and equestrian sports. Through the Development Assistance Programme of the FEI, National Federations are encouraged to seek help from other federations which may be able to provide particular expertise.

The FEI in conjunction with National Federations promotes scientific studies of equine health. Results are available to National Federations which are responsible for distribution as appropriate, for example the *Stress in Travel* booklet.

(7) In the interests of the horse, the fitness and competence of the rider or driver shall be regarded as essential.

In all equestrian sports, at every level, the ability of a horse's partner has a direct bearing on its well-being and performance. The horse must be athletically trained for the purpose for which it is being used. It is equally important that the rider is suitably fit and competent for that purpose in order to assist the horse to perform to the best of its ability; an unfit rider may hinder the horse.

(8) All training methods should take account of the horse as a living creature and must not include any technique considered by the FEI to be abusive.

At all times when a horse is being trained or used in competition its physiological and psychological make-up should be considered. It is important to take into account how the horse's body works and how its mental attitude and fitness affect its performance. At no time should equipment such as whips, spurs, bits and reins be used in such a way as to cause pain or injury.

(9) National Federations must establish adequate controls in order that all persons and bodies under their jurisdiction respect the welfare of the horse.

National Federations are responsible for ensuring that their rules and regulations adequately safeguard the welfare of horses. These rules must be rigorously enforced by a suitable judicial system so that disciplinary action can be taken against those who transgress them. Where possible the rules and regulations should mirror those of the FEI.

(10) Rules regarding the health and welfare of horses must be strictly adhered to, not only in competition, but also in training. Such rules and regulations shall be regularly reviewed.

The rules of national competition, by being similar to those of the FEI, ensure that the same high standards of care and welfare apply. As equestrian sport develops it is important that the rules protect the horse from undue pressure. In due course experience will necessitate refinement of the existing rules and the introduction of new ones. Legislation must be introduced to counteract any emerging practices which are contrary to the welfare of the horse.

Index